Irene Kassor

Color Atlas of

CRITICAL AND INTENSIVE CARE
Diagnosis and Investigation

David W Ryan MB ChB FRCA
Director of Intensive Care
Freeman Hospital
Newcastle upon Tyne
UK

Gilbert R Park MD MA FRCA
Director of Intensive Care
Addenbrooke's Hospital
Cambridge
UK

M Mosby-Wolfe

London Baltimore Bogotá Boston Buenos Aires Caracas Carlsbad, CA Chicago Madrid Mexico City Milan Naples, FL New York Philadelphia St. Louis Sydney Tokyo Toronto Wiesbaden

Copyright © 1995 Times Mirror International Publishers Limited

Published in 1995 by Mosby-Wolfe, an imprint of Times Mirror International
Publishers Limited

Printed by Grafos S.A. Arte sobre papel, Barcelona, Spain

ISBN 0 7234 1956 6

For full details of all Times Mirror International Publishers Limited titles,
please write to Times Mirror International Publishers Limited, Lynton House,
7–12 Tavistock Square, London WC1H 9LB, England.

A CIP catalogue record for this book is available from the British Library.

Library of Congress Cataloging-in-Publication Data applied for.

Project Manager:	Peter Harrison
Developmental Editor:	Claire Hooper/Lucy Hamilton
Designer/Layout Artist:	Lara Last
Cover Design:	Ian Spick
Illustration:	Marion Tusker
Production:	Mike Heath
Index:	Dr Laurence Errington
Publisher:	Geoff Greenwood

Contents

To Susan for her continuing support *DWR*
To Nikon and Kodak for giving me the tools *GRP*

INTRODUCTION

This Atlas is designed for nurses, doctors, medical students, allied professions, representatives from industry and non-specialist medical trainees who want to learn more about intensive care. It avoids paediatrics, the exotic and on the whole the uncommon, unless a point is to be made. It offers a simple approach to a most complex subject.

When we started planning this book we wondered where to stop. Intensive care medicine encompasses all areas of medicine, and we could have written an Atlas of enormous size. We decided not to do this — it would have ben prohibitively expensive in any case. We have therefore included only a small proportion of what was possible. Hopefully it includes the most important and interesting aspects of intensive care medicine.

One early reviewer commented that no-one would want to look at pictures of patients on machines. We agree. The technology is a means to an end. We hope this book looks beyond that initial impression, prevents the inevitable shut-off that follows and allows assessment by means of clinical signs, a practical approach with understanding of the conditions encountered, and most of all common sense in dealing with the treatment of the critically ill.

ACKNOWLEDGEMENTS

Permission was obtained from all the staff, patients and/or relatives who appear in photographs used in this Atlas. The majority of these photographs have been masked, but where they are not consent was obtained.

Many clinicians contributed their ideas, advice and expert comments, and offered their slides to illustrate conditions in this Atlas. We thank them all. Dr Leslie Lai gave advice on the biochemical values.

Hospital Update gave permission to reproduce slides from previously published articles by both authors. These were: Figs 9; 22; 24; 35; 36; 40; 41; 49; 61; 70; 114; 115; 130; 372; 374; 378; 385.

The majority of slides were taken by the Departments of Medical Illustration, University of Cambridge and University of Newcastle upon Tyne.

The following illustrations are reproduced by permission of Dr T. Ashcroft, Fig. 275; Dr M. Bennett, Figs 46, 57, 60, 108, 195, 253, 274, 326, 329, 341, 354, 417, 418; Mr J. Chamberlain, Figs 25, 29–32, 39, 178; Dr I. Conacher, Figs 263, 264; Dr N. Cooper, Fig. 402; Department of Medical Physics, Freeman Hospital, Figs 331–334, 344, 413; Dr S. Elliott, Figs 106, 319, 320, 321, 416; Professor J. Gibson and Respiratory Laboratories, Freeman Hospital, Figs 255, 256, 261, 262; Dr K. Gould, Figs 434, 445–449; Dr S. Hunter, Figs 337, 338; Dr D. Kapur, Figs 397–399; Dr P. Kestervan, Figs 440–444; Dr L. Lai, Fig. 407; Mr M. Lennard, Figs 267–268; Dr H. Loose, Fig. 102; Professor D. Mendelow, Figs 162 and 163; Mr D. Meikle, Figs 202, 203; Dr L. Mitchell, Figs 327, 328; Dr A. Morley Fig. 105; Dr B. Nicholls, Fig. 144; Mr I. Pinder, Figs 10, 426; Dr H. Powell, Fig. 389; Mr P. Ramsden, Fig. 429; Dr J. Rose, Figs 94 and 95; Mr R. Sengupta, Figs 159–161; SSI Ltd, Figs 223, 224; Dr A. Soni, Fig. 249; Dr C. Tilbury Figs 34, 152, 153; Dr P. Tjong Joe-Wai, Fig. 8; Dr B. Watson, Fig. 248; Professor R. Wilkinson, Figs 325, 427; Dr Zammit Maepel, Fig. 419.

Figs 54, 154, 322, and 432 are reproduced with permission from *A Colour Atlas and Text of Clinical Medicine*, C.D. Forbes and W.F. Jackson, Mosby-Year Book Europe, London, 1993. Fig. 164 is reproduced with permission from Vol. 1 of *A Colour Atlas of Chest Trauma*, A. Besson and F. Saegesser, Wolfe Medical Publications, London, 1982.

Figs 356 and 357 are reproduced by permission of the European Resuscitation Council and the Resuscitation Council (UK), and are available from Laerdal Medical Ltd.

Chapter 1 Clinical conditions and physical signs

CLINICAL CONDITIONS

ACUTE RESPIRATORY DISTRESS

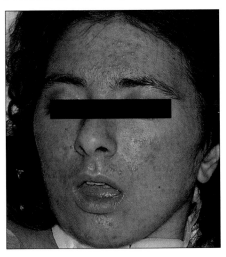

Fig. 1 Characteristically the facies appear vacant, the brow is furrowed in concentration, and covered in sweat. The *alar nasae* are flared with the lips parted and cyanosed in this patient. The respiratory rate is increasing and over 40 breaths a minute. The appearance is one of a desperate struggle to stay alive.

The definition of respiratory failure is a pH >7.35 or H^+ = 45 nmol/l, a PaO_2 < 8 kPa on air and a $PaCO_2$ >6.7 kPa. Sometimes forgotten is the fourth component of this definition, a respiratory rate exceeding 35 breaths per min. This is an important reason for admission to the ICU. Mechanical ventilation is life saving.

SHOCK

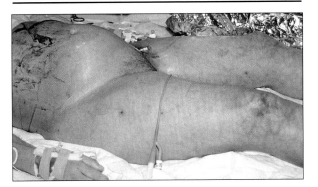

Fig. 2 The limbs are poorly perfused and cyanosed. Shock is circulatory failure characterised by inadequate oxygen delivery to the tissues. Death is common unless the condition is recognised and the downward spiral stopped. This obstetric patient had a precipitous decrease in blood pressure after a post-partum haemorrhage.

CYANOSIS

Fig. 3 Cyanosis is present in this nail bed, indicating a level of reduced haemoglobin of at least 5 g/dl. Central causes include abnormal haemoglobins, chronic lung disease, polycythaemia and massive pulmonary embolism. Peripheral cyanosis is due to the cold, circulatory failure or peripheral vascular disease.

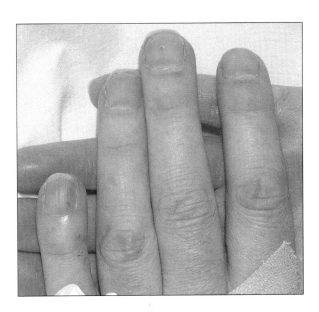

SURGICAL EMPHYSEMA

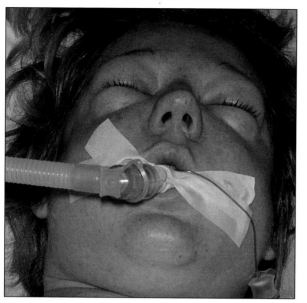

Fig. 4 The orbits are blown up with air as this picture shows. This woman developed generalised surgical emphysema secondary to asthma, producing a 'Michelin man' appearance. Surgical emphysema is readily diagnosed by a crackling sensation under the skin on palpation. Fractured ribs, chest or neck surgery are other frequent causes.

TRAUMA

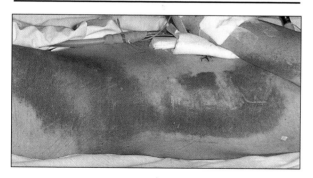

Fig. 6 Haematoma often drains posteriorly and may not be seen unless looked for. This man was admitted after an assault. A brutal injury can result in abdominal injury and massive blood loss. Assessing the degree of blood loss after trauma is difficult. The priorities include achieving a mean arterial pressure of 70 mmHg, an SpO_2 >90% and an adequate urine output >1 ml/kg/h.

BURN

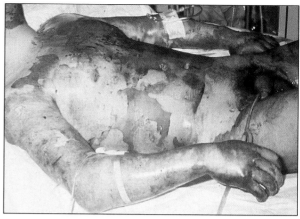

Fig. 5 The three degrees of burn injury are shown in this house-fire victim.

Careful mapping is needed to distinguish a first-degree burn of the epidermis with erythema and pain, a second degree burn with painful sensation and blistering down to the dermis and a third degree burn with death of all skin layers, no sensation and a leathery texture. In adults the extent of a burn injury is mapped using a 'rule of nines'. The anterior and posterior surfaces of each leg, each arm, and the head are estimated to contain 9% of the body surface area, the anterior and posterior thorax contain 18% respectively, and the perineum 1%; for a child allow 14% for the head but only 16% for each leg.

CELLULITIS

Fig. 7 This arm shows a nasty weeping cellulitis. This labourer had had a minimal injury at work and was admitted with a temperature over 40°C. It can be a life-threatening infection requiring treatment in the ICU.

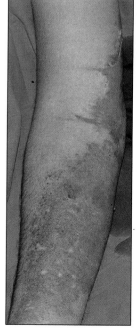

DRUG ADDICT

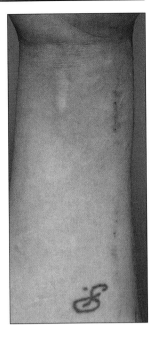

Fig. 8 Numerous scars from venepunctures along with thrombosis of the veins are seen along the arm. A drainage site of a former infected abscess is also shown at the wrist. This patient was 'mainlining' heroin. Drug addicts are at a particular risk when in the ICU. They may be carriers of the hepatitis B virus (the risk is increased by tattooing) and HIV infection.

FAT EMBOLISM

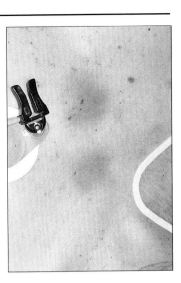

Fig. 9 Petechia over chest after long bone fractures consistent with fat emboli. The bruising may also have occurred at the time of injury but also could have been produced by doctors squeezing the skin to elicit a pain response.

MULTIPLE INJURY: VOLKMANN'S ISCHAEMIC CONTRACTURE

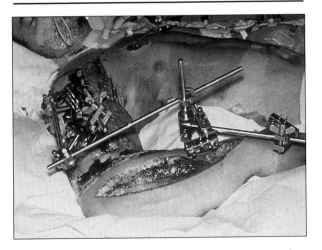

Fig. 10 Circulatory impairment can occur after supracondylar fractures because of damage to the brachial artery. The surgeon has performed a fasciotomy to relieve pressure around the artery. It must be looked for carefully in all multiply-injured patients with this fracture, especially if they are unconscious.

COMPARTMENT SYNDROME

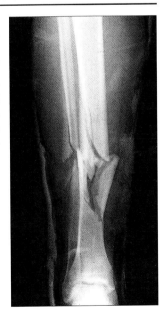

Fig. 11 Bleeding into the muscles of the leg after a fracture has resulted in a critical compression of the circulation. Prompt removal of a restricting Plaster of Paris cast and fasciotomies is required to restore the circulation and save the leg.

PETECHIA

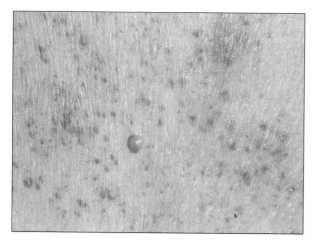

Fig. 12 Numerous small petechia are seen over the abdomen. This is an accompaniment of thrombocytopenia and in this patient suggested the disseminated intravascular coagulation (DIC) syndrome. DIC is associated with increased bleeding caused by consumption of the clotting factors, activation of the fibrinolytic syndrome and thrombosis. The causes of DIC are multiple, but include sepsis, obstetric catastrophes, vascular disorders, malignant disease, and massive tissue injury.

PITTING OEDEMA

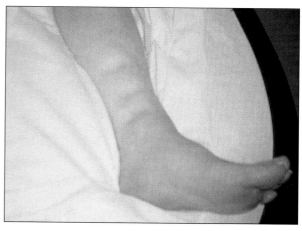

Fig. 13 Gross oedema, as shown in this picture, may be the result of cardiac, hepatic or renal failure, and nutritional impairment (low albumin). Unilateral oedema is the result of a venous thrombosis or lymphatic obstruction, e.g. malignancy, parasite, or after venous or arterial cannulation of the limb.

JAUNDICE

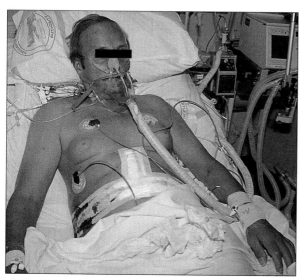

Fig. 14 Jaundice is clinically evident when the serum bilirubin exceeds 50 μmol/l. It has many causes. In the critically ill patient sepsis, viral infections and drugs are common causes. Some patients may abruptly develop fulminant hepatic failure, leading to encephalopathy, coagulopathy, and renal failure. Sepsis, gastrointestinal haemorrhage, aspiration pneumonia, respiratory failure and cerebral oedema are common complications.

ANAEMIA

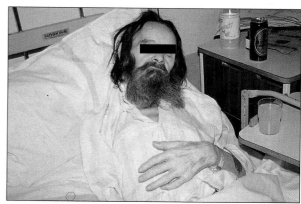

Fig. 15 This patient has a haemoglobin concentration of 5.5 g/dl caused by bleeding from the bladder. He is extremely pale.

FLUID EXTRAVASATION

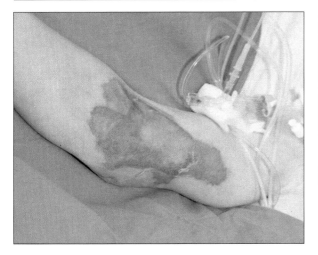

Fig. 16 This angry-looking and blistering elbow and arm resulted from an infusion of fluid under pressure. The infusion 'tissued' and unfortunately this went unnoticed.

URAEMIA

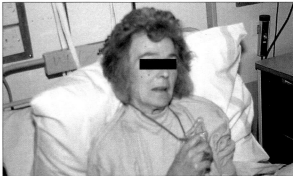

Fig. 17 This lady's sallow appearance is due to long-standing uraemia secondary to chronic renal failure. Her urea blood is 60 mmol/l (normal 2.5–7 mmol/l) with a creatinine of 630 mmol/l (normal 65–110 mmol/l) despite haemodialysis three times a week.

EXTERNAL PHYSICAL SIGNS

SACRAL PRESSURE SORE

The incidence of pressure sores is at least 7% in all hospital patients. It is a common finding when patients are admitted to the ICU. The commonest sites are at the sacrum, trochanter and heel areas.
Fig. 18 This stage 4 sore (see **Table 1** below) is deceptive, as the cavity looks small. The actual area of necrosis is much larger and some impression of this is given by the inflammatory circle around the ulcer.

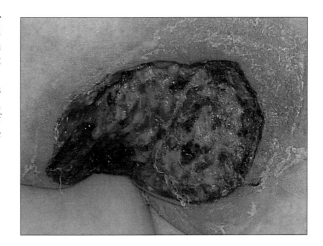

Table 1 Staging pressure sores

Stage 1	Nonblanchable erythema
Stage 2	Partial thickness skin loss involving epidermis or dermis. Superficial abrasion, blister or shallow ulcer
Stage 3	Full thickness skin loss, damage or necrosis down to, but not through, underlying facia. Presents as a deep ulcer
Stage 4	Full thickness skin loss with extensive destruction

SUPERFICIAL BLISTERS

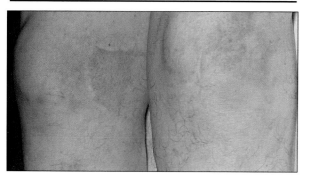

Fig. 19 Blisters can be caused by drug reactions, dermatitis herpetiformis and pemphigoid.

PRESSURE SORE TO HEEL

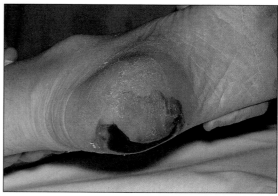

Fig. 20 Stage 3 sore (see **Table 1**, p. 9).

SCALP PRESSURE SORE

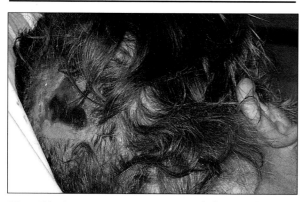

Fig. 21 A pressure sore caused by prolonged immobility after coma. Small, sick infants are particularly prone to this complication if they are not picked up or moved about.

CHICKENPOX

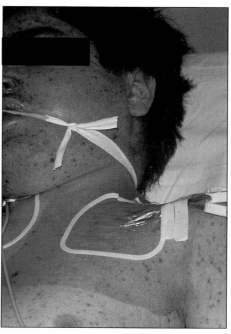

Fig. 22 The classic distribution of the vesicular rash is central, with crops appearing over a few days. Chickenpox is a particular risk in patients with an altered immune system. It is highly infectious. The respiratory tract and lungs are often affected.

ACUTE PSORIASIS

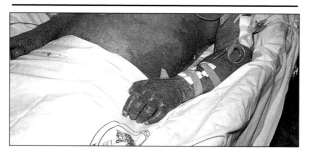

Fig. 23 This patient's psoriasis has been aggravated by stopping the normal treatment given during a period of severe illness.

RHEUMATOID BRUISING

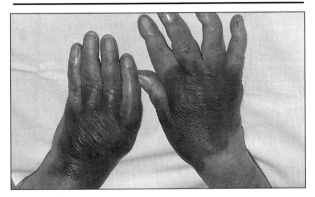

Fig. 24 This patient with classical rheumatoid arthritis of the hands had a single clean venepuncture in each hand with a resulting substantial bruise. The steroids the patient had received over a period of time contributed to this process.

DIABETIC FOOT

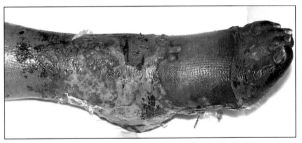

Fig. 25 This foot is chronically infected; it is covered in pustules and the toes are gangrenous. Care of the feet is a major challenge in diabetes mellitus patients, who are also prone to peripheral vascular disease. These patients often present in the ICU after some complications of their disease have occurred or after surgery.

FOOT DROP

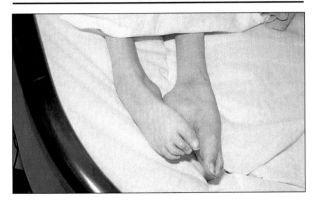

Fig. 26 Failure to provide proper physiotherapy on a daily basis resulted in prolonged foot drop in this trauma case. Six months after discharge this had not resolved.

EMBOLISM TO FINGER

Fig. 27 This isch-aemia to the index finger followed in-sertion of an arterial line. A continuous heparin flush had been omitted. Small emboli formed and embolised the tip of this finger.

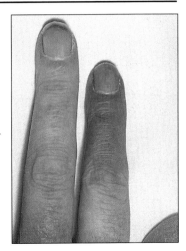

WEGNER'S GRANULOMA: AFFECTING THE NOSE

Fig. 28 This patient presented to the ICU with a typical granu-lomatous lesion of the nose. The hands and lungs are also affected. A severe glomerulonephritis occurs.

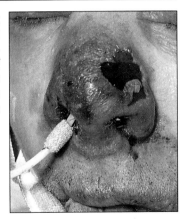

WHITE LEG

Fig. 29 An acute embolus has been thrown off from the heart, causing total inter-ruption of the arterial cir-culation to the foot. An ischaemic toe suggestive of pre-existing peripheral vas-cular disease is present.

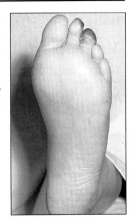

PAINFUL ISCHAEMIA OF FOOT

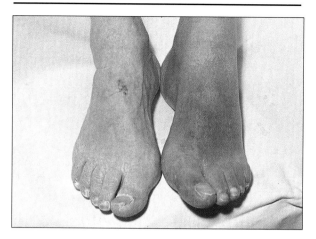

Fig. 30 The characteristic hyperaemia on the dorsum of the foot suggests compromised circulation, with a cyanosed great toe area which is already ischaemic. Avoid cannulation in this foot.

DEEP VEIN THROMBOSIS

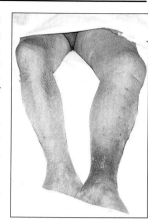

Fig. 31 The left leg is swollen and painful. The patient also has an ischaemic foot. The majority of venous thromboses arise in the veins of the pelvis and the leg. Low-dose heparin and compression stockings are an effective combination to prevent venous thrombosis prophylactically, and should be used routinely in the ICU setting.

VENOGRAM OF PELVIC VEIN

Fig. 32 A thrombus (arrow) is easily visualised in the right iliac vein on venography. Surgery, trauma, orthopaedic procedures, pelvic surgery, prolonged immobility, congestive heart failure, COPD, pregnancy, obesity, malignancy and the oestrogen-containing contraceptive pill are just some of the diverse predisposing conditions putting patients at risk.

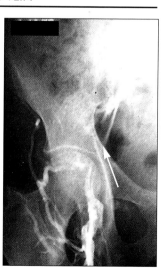

HERPES SIMPLEX OF THE EYES AND NOSE

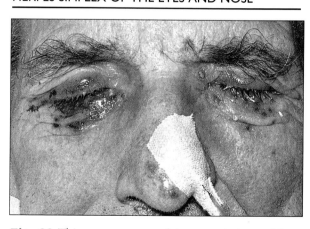

Fig. 33 This case occurred in association with a pneumococcal pneumonia. It is important that an ophthalmologist is asked to advise on management. Failure to do this may result in permanent corneal damage.

SNAKE BITE

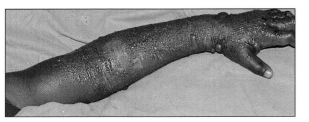

Fig. 34 An unidentified snake bite showing extensive oedema involving the whole arm and extending onto the chest wall. A cause of DIC.

ERYTHEMA MULTIFORMA

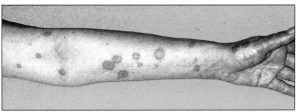

Fig. 35 Classical target lesions distributed peripherally caused by a herpes simplex infection.

IATROGENIC SKIN DAMAGE

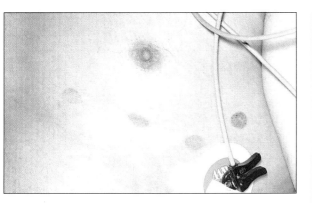

Fig. 36 Attachment of skin electrodes has resulted in these skin lesions.

'TRASH' FOOT

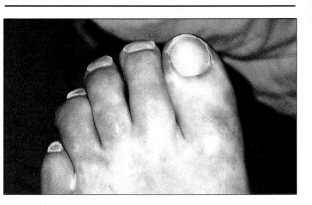

Fig. 38 Small thrombi have showered down the peripheral vessels during surgery giving this typical appearance of distal ischaemia.

INTRA-ARTERIAL TEMAZEPAM

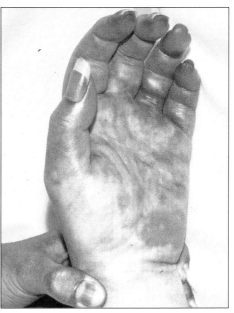

Fig. 37 Gangrene of the hand. A self-administered intra-arterial injection of temazepam. Amputation was necessary. Similar results may follow accidental arterial injection of drugs such as phenytoin, flucloxacillin and thiopentone.

COLD INJURY

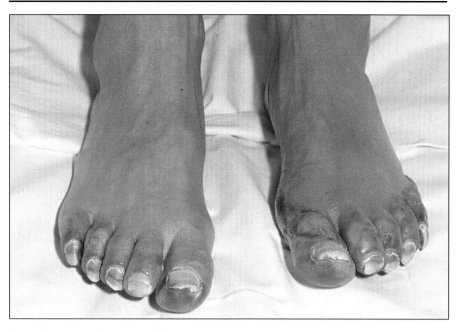

Fig. 39 The combination of freezing tissue and extreme arterial vasoconstriction leads to permanent damage. Seen here is the hyperaemic response that causes a 'pumpkin hue' adjacent to gangrenous toes as the feet rewarm. It is important to treat this injury at the same time as the patient with profound hypothermia is being rewarmed to minimise longer-term disability to the feet.

INTRAVENOUS ADRENALINE

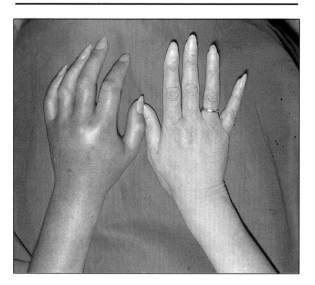

Fig. 40 Adrenaline and other inotropic drugs given through a peripheral line (in this case at a cardiac arrest situation) may produce profound vaso-constriction to the limb. Inotropic agents, when possible, should always be given via a central line by an infusion pump.

EXTRAVASATION OF BICARBONATE

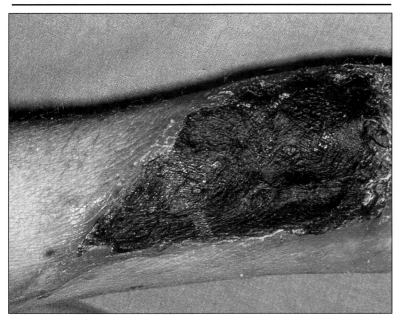

Fig. 41 In this case sodium bicarbonate has extravasated causing local gangrene. Drugs used in resuscitation can cause major damage when given via peripheral veins.

CALCIUM DEPOSITS

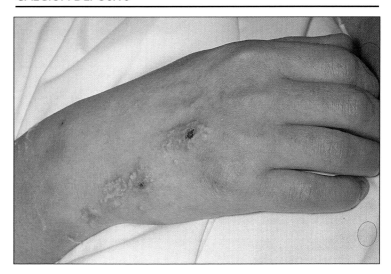

Fig. 42 Ten ml of intravenous calcium gluconate given at a cardiac arrest resulted in permanent calcified foci along the line of the vein. Calcified deposits like this are often seen in other conditions such as chronic renal failure.

SEPSIS

INTRODUCTION

Sepsis is the most common complication in the ICU. Community and nosocomial infections are equally common as the source of infection. Factors such as diabetes mellitus, surgery of the gastrointestinal tract and altered immune status predispose the patient to infection. The classical features of sepsis are hyperventilation, confusion , a high temperature, rigors, a warm periphery and an increasing white cell count. In 15% of cases the septic shock syndrome develops, with profound hypotension, DIC and renal failure; this is associated with a mortality of 75%. Generalised sepsis leads to multiorgan failure.

CARDIOVASCULAR CHANGES IN SEVERE SEPSIS

Table 2 shows typical values of deranged cardiovascular parameters (see **Table 9** and **Table 10**, p. 53, for a detailed discussion) from a case of septicaemia caused by *Escherichia coli* isolated from the blood and sputum of this patient following bowel surgery.

There is a high cardiac output (CO) (normal 4–8 l/min), a low systemic vascular resistance (SVR) (normal 1440 dyne/s/cm^{-5}) resulting in a low mean arterial pressure (MAP). The oxygen delivery ($\dot{D}O_2I$) is adequate at 907 (normal >600 ml/min/m^2) but the oxygen consumption ($\dot{V}O_2I$) is also markedly increased at 227 (normal >167 ml/min/m^2). The patient was treated with antibiotics, and an infusion of phenylephidrine. The haemoglobin was increased with a blood transfusion. A subphrenic collection (see **Fig. 52**, p. 18) was confirmed by CT scan and drained.

Table 3 shows the situation 24 hours later. The patient is stable but the oxygen consumption continues to increase, indicating the septic state was not under control.

SEPTIC SHOCK SYNDROME

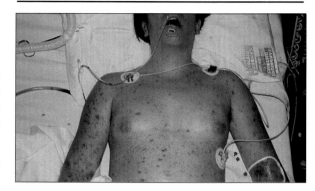

Fig. 43 The clinical picture is usually obvious. The presence of sepsis is not synonymous with bacteria, as any organism can cause this condition. Gram-negative organisms account for 80% of bacterial sepsis in the ICU, but it is impossible clinically to distinguish from Gram-positive infection. Note the purpuric rash caused by DIC.

Table 2 Severe sepsis (1)

Input values				
MAP	77	mmHg	PaO_2	10.6 kPa
CVP	7	mmHg	SaO_2	90%
MPAP	26	mmHg	$S\bar{v}O_2$	73%
PCWP	8	mmHg	Hb	10.09 g/dl

Calculated values				
AVG	CO	9.51	CaO_2 (97)	14.4
AVG	CI	6.3	$C\bar{v}O_2$ (73)	10.8
BSA		1.99	$\dot{D}O_2I$	907
SVR		588	$\dot{V}O_2I$	227
SVRI		904		

Table 3 Severe sepsis (2); 24 hours later

Input values				
MAP	74	mmHg	PaO_2	12kPa
CVP	12	mmHg	SaO_2	95%
MPAP	26	mmHg	$S\bar{v}O_2$	73%
PCWP	9	mmHg	Hb	12.1 g/dl

Calculated values				
AVG	CO	8.25	CaO_2 (95)	16.5
AVG	CI	5.50	$C\bar{v}O_2$ (67)	11.4
BSA		1.50	$\dot{D}O_2I$	908
SVR		601	$\dot{V}O_2I$	281
SVRI		895		

MAXILLARY SINUS ABSCESS

Fig. 44 This malar flush, which also suggests mitral valve disease, was hot to the touch.

This is a dangerous infection of the maxillary sinus, resulting in a cavernous vein thrombosis. This patient had gangrene of the nose from a previous naso-tracheal tube and this caused the infection.

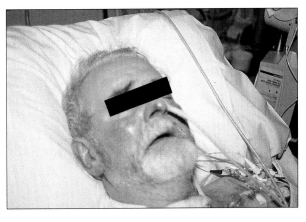

SEPTIC EMBOLI: OSLER'S NODES

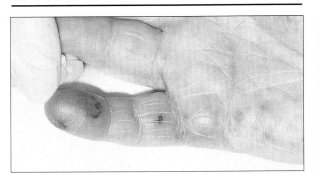

Fig. 45 These painful infarcted fingertips are secondary to septic emboli resulting from vegetations on the heart valves caused by subacute bacterial endocarditis (SBE).

CATHETER DAMAGE LEADING TO BACTERIAL ENDOCARDITIS

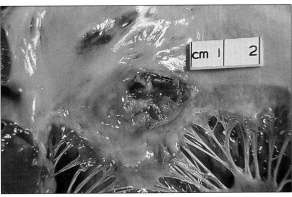

Fig. 46 Right-sided central catheters and pulmonary artery catheters (PACs) can damage the heart. They can also seed infection. An incidence of SBE as high as 7% following their use has been quoted. This is sometimes missed in the critically ill and highlights the need to investigate all new heart murmurs in such patients.

PARONYCHIA

Fig. 47 A pulp-space infection of the nailbed occurred after pruning roses. The patient needed admission to the ICU to treat an overwhelming staphylococcal infection. All such patients need to be carefully examined for small lesions of this kind. The source of the illness can then often be identified.

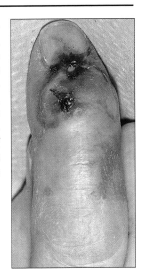

GAS GANGRENE

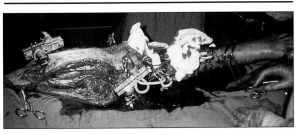

Fig. 48 This man was dragged behind a delivery van. *Clostridia perfringens* was isolated from the leg wound. His leg had to be amputated to prevent further deterioration. He developed renal failure, but eventually recovered.

MENINGOCOCCAL MENINGITIS

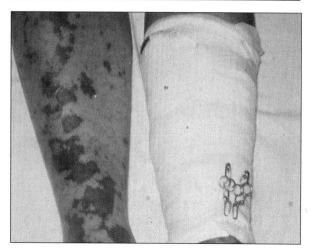

Fig. 49 The classic development of haemorrhagic areas over the skin within hours of developing meningococcal septicaemia is shown here.

ABSCESS OF LIVER

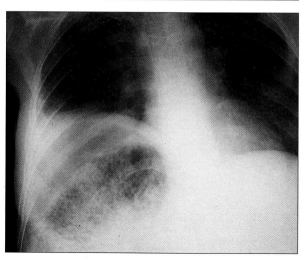

Fig. 50 A gas-forming organism was responsible for this unique radiographic appearance. Liver abscess is a known infective complication of liver transplantation, as in this case. Bacterial abscesses are uncommon, which is surprising in view of the frequency of cholangitis, peritonitis and bowel infections as a source of infection.

Abscesses occur in the liver with *Entamoeba histolytica* infections and this needs exclusion in certain parts of the world where this is endemic or after holidays in such regions.

PERSISTENT INFECTION

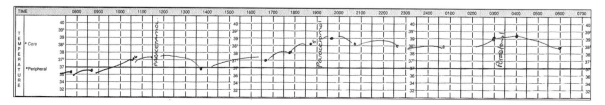

Fig. 51 This temperature chart shows repeated periods of undulating temperature over 24 hours. This continued for 14 days. Rigorous attempts to identify the source may be necessary including bronchial washings, repeated cultures of blood, CSF, sinus washings, urine and faeces, ultrasound of the abdomen, transoesophageal echocardiography of the heart and CT scanning. All venous and arterial access lines should be removed and sent for culture.

CT SCAN OF SUBPHRENIC COLLECTION

Fig. 52 A subphrenic collection (arrow) is a particular risk after biliary and bowel perforation. The condition occurs less frequently since the advent of improved surgical techniques, and especially of prophylactic antibiotics aimed at the anaerobic group of organisms. Confirmation and percutaneous drainage can be made with an ultrasound or CT scan. This makes further surgery unnecessary for some patients.

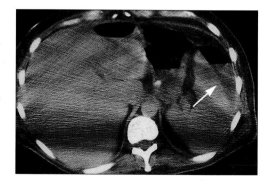

THE IMMUNOCOMPROMISED PATIENT

Patients with altered immune status are increasingly being admitted to the ICU with infection. The majority of these cases fall into patient groups associated with transplantation, chemotherapy, malignancy, acquired immune deficiency syndrome (AIDS), lengthy steroid treatment or after splenectomy. In the ICU such patients need to be barrier-nursed in positive-inflow cubicles as they present such a high risk of contracting infections.

Gram-negative, staphylococcal, fungal and yeast infections are the most likely causes of sepsis. In such patients there is a much greater likelihood of less common organisms, and a persistent fever should always lead to consideration of fungal infections. Strenuous efforts should be made to isolate the source of the infection (see **Fig. 58**, p. 20).

HERPES SIMPLEX OF THE LEG

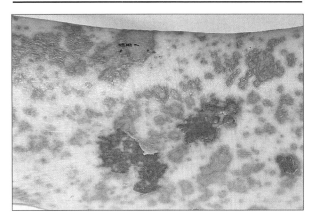

Fig. 53 Systemic herpes simplex infections can occur as a life-threatening disease in immunocompromised patients. Here it has occurred following a renal transplant.

CANDIDA INFECTION OF THE MOUTH

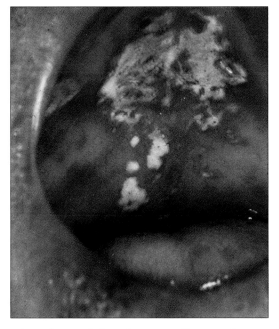

Fig. 54 *Candida* infections affecting the mouth in acute leukaemia and after transplantation are common. Some groups are routinely given oral antifungal agents to prevent this.

CANDIDA OF THE OESOPHAGUS

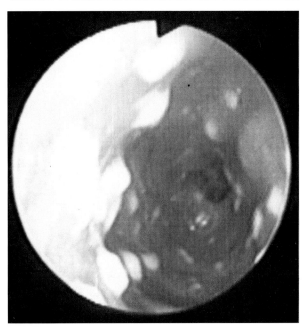

Fig. 55 The oesophagus is affected in this case of gastric cancer. Nystatin mouth washes usually control the infection locally. Systemic infections are difficult to treat.

ASPERGILLOSIS

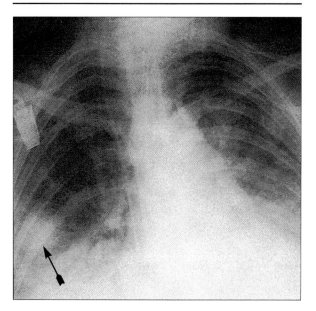

Fig. 56 Aspergillosis must be suspected when this typical cavity appearance (arrow) is seen on a chest radiograph. The diagnosis usually needs a bronchial lavage or open lung biopsy.

ASPERGILLOMA: LUNG

Fig. 57 Systemic treatment with amphotericin is required as soon as the diagnosis is confirmed. Survival beyond 2–3 weeks is uncommon in the neutropenic patient. This postmortem specimen was removed from a patient who had died with disseminated aspergillosis.

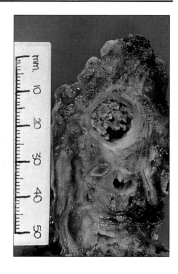

BRONCHIAL LAVAGE

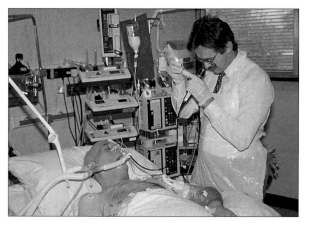

Fig. 58 This is a diagnostic procedure in the ICU. It can be undertaken in patients requiring ventilatory support cases. Around 60 ml of 0.9% normal saline are instilled down each main bronchus in turn and aspirated into a sterile container. The laboratory should be alerted to expect the sample. The use of blind 'protected tip' endobronchial catheters will soon replace this procedure.

OPEN LUNG BIOPSY

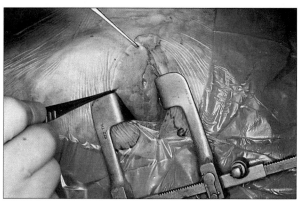

Fig. 59 The alternative procedure to bronchial lavage is open lung biopsy, by its nature a more major undertaking. Samples should be sent for both histology and microbiology.

PNEUMOCYSTIS CARINII: LUNG

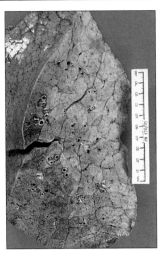

Fig. 60 This is especially common in AIDS patients. There is often little in the way of symptoms apart from increasing dyspnoea. Measurement of arterial blood gases often shows severe hypoxia. Early treatment has resulted in a dramatic fall in the mortality of this condition. High dose trimethoprim, sometimes with pentamidine, is used.

KAPOSI'S SARCOMA

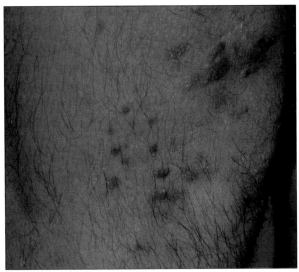

Fig. 61 This is a neoplastic process occurring in AIDS patients. These patients may present with a severe pneumonia.

CYTOMEGALIC VIRUS (CMV)

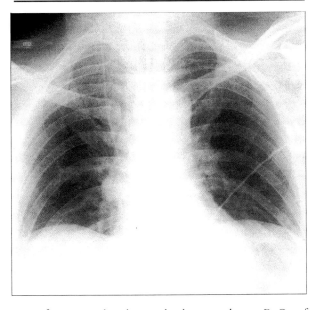

Fig. 62 Minimal radiograph changes, but a PaO_2 of 4 kPa on air led to suspicion of an opportunistic infection. Bronchial lavage in this patient who had had a renal transplant revealed cytomegalic virus (CMV) infection. This is transmitted to transplant patients by blood transfusion and the transplanted organ.

LEGIONNAIRE'S DISEASE

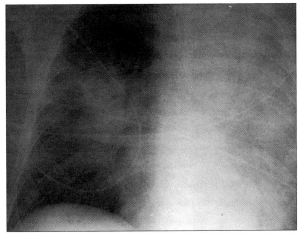

Fig. 63 A left bronchopneumonia and right lobar pneumonia. This man returning from holiday in Spain had a prodromal history of cough and malaise, diarrhoea with some nausea and vomiting and recent chest pain before admission. He had a PaO_2 of 4.9 kPa on room air with a $PaCO_2$ of 5.5 kPa. He was alert and talking. Mechanical ventilation on 100% oxygen only improved the PaO_2 to 8 kPa. To make the diagnosis bronchial lavage was necessary.

FLORID ACNE

Fig. 64 Outbreaks of *Staphylococcus* skin infections are seen in ICU patients. This patient had a flare-up of her acne during a prolonged illness.

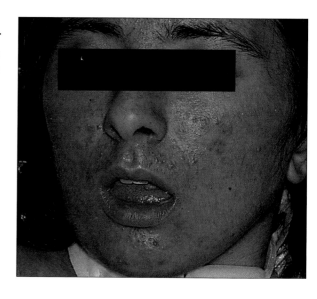

ASSESSING NUTRITION

Inadequate nutrition is a feature of illness. Patients may have suffered anorexia, diarrhoea or vomiting before their admission. The influence of injury results in a catabolic process that causes muscle cannibalism. A weight loss of 10% is significant. In a similar fashion, a sudden increase in weight suggests fluid retention. The nutritional needs of patients vary, but all need a combination of water, electrolytes, vitamins, trace elements, carbohydrate, protein and fat. Failure to provide adequate nutrition exposes the patients to infection, poor wound healing, muscle wasting and lessens their chances of survival.

GROSS OBESITY

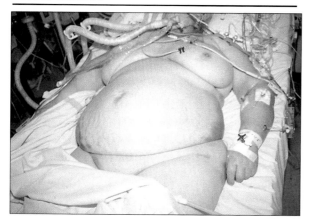

Fig. 65 Massive obesity is an increasing feature of the Western diet. Such enormity compromises respiration, and is often accompanied by reduced central respiratory drive. Surgery is likely to aggravate the problems. Immobility, deep vein thrombosis, poor venous access, poor hygiene and an immense nursing task are some of the problems of dealing with these cases.

ANOREXIA NERVOSA

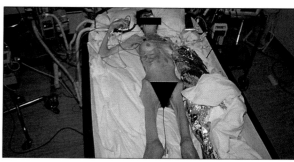

Fig. 66 This 26-year-old woman collapsed on the way home from work. Her blood sugar was <2 mmol/l (normal 4–6 mmol/l), and her lack of body mass meant she had no energy reserve. She gave a history of refusing to eat that day, leading to this hypoglycaemic attack.

CATABOLISM

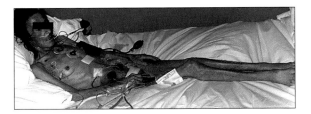

Fig. 67 This 43-year-old woman was admitted with multiple abdominal fistulas and sepsis, pressure sores and a body weight of 30 kg. A year previously she had undergone radiation for cancer of the cervix and had subsequently developed radiation ileus. She died as a result of wasting of the cardiac and respiratory muscles.

FLUIDISED BED

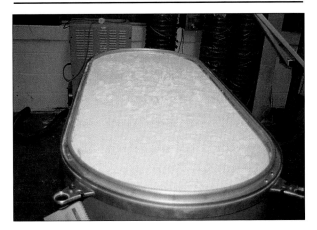

Fig. 68 Nursing patients in a cocoon of warm air at 32°C has been shown to reduce nitrogen losses by 4 g/24 hours and caloric usage by 400–600 cal per day. The bed also permits ease of handling of extremes of body build, permits weighing of the patient, and reduces pain and the stress response.

ASSESSING NUTRITION

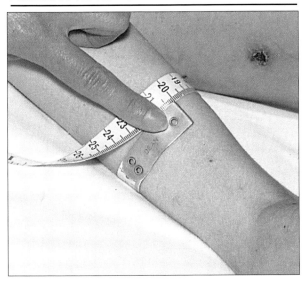

Fig. 69 Anthropomorphic measurements (pictured here) are more useful in research. Serial weight changes need to be coupled with the measurement of serum albumin, white blood cell count and 24-hour urine collections (to measure 80% of nitrogen losses as urinary urea) to provide a picture of the patient's nutritional position (see **Fig. 405**, p. 121). Recently it has become possible to measure the metabolic rate at the bedside, but it has limited accuracy when the F_IO_2 exceeds 0.5, which it is likely to be in the majority of critically ill patients. The use of formulas based on age, weight, height and energy expenditure is favoured by dieticians, who may overestimate requirements, whilst doctors tend to underestimate them.

ENTERAL FEEDING: FINE BORE TUBE

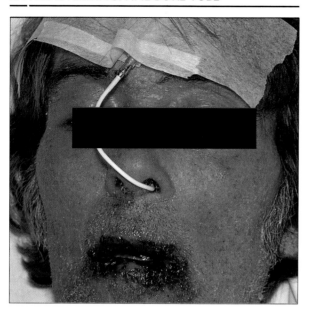

Fig. 70 The easiest and safest method of feeding is to use the gut. This patient with Stevens-Johnson syndrome (see **Figs 120** and **121**, p. 36) has a fine bore tube inserted. This replaces a large bore nasogastric tube when the patient has started to absorb fluids.

FINE BORE TUBE IN LUNG

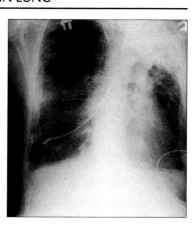

Fig. 71 It is easy to insert a fine bore tube into the lungs incorrectly. Infusion of feed can lead to inflammation, chest infection and lung collapse. Before starting the feed check the position of the feeding tube on a chest radiograph.

PUMP FEEDING

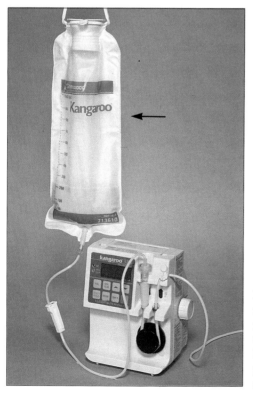

NASAL GASTROENTEROSTOMY TUBE

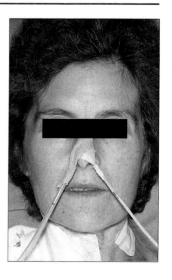

Fig. 73 This woman has both a nasogastric (right) and gastroenterostomy tube (left) present.

Fig. 72 The milky-looking sterile feed (arrow) is infused by a dedicated pump located directly beneath it. A break in 24-hour continuous feeding must be made to prevent colonisation of the stomach by bacteria with a corresponding increase in nosocomial pneumonia. This also allows aspiration of the stomach to ensure it is emptying.

ENTERAL FEEDING: GASTROENTEROSTOMY TUBE

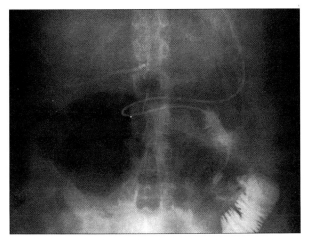

Fig. 74 The frequent handicap of postoperative gastric ileus is overcome by this simple procedure.

AN ABDOMINAL GASTROENTEROSTOMY TUBE

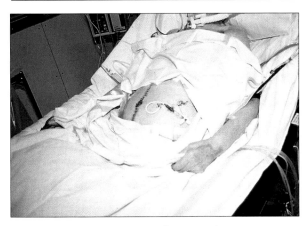

Fig. 75 Feeding can start 36 hours after surgery.

GROSS FAECAL LOADING

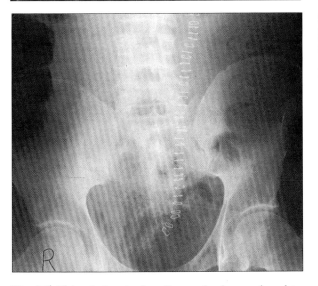

Fig. 76 This abdominal radiograph shows the skin clips along the wound and gross faecal loading from the rectum to one-third of the way along the transverse colon. Constipation is a not unusual finding in ill patients and is aggravated by the widespread use of opioids and other sedative agents.

PERIPHERAL VEIN TPN

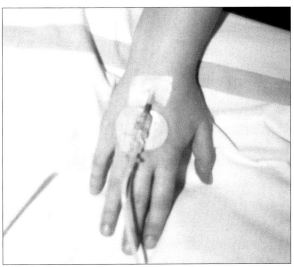

Fig. 77 In some circumstances peripheral vein TPN can provide a useful interim measure. To preserve the vein a useful trick is to place a nitrate patch distal (not proximal) to the intravenous site.

PARENTERAL NUTRITION

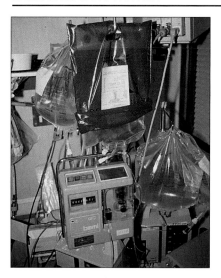

Fig. 78 In the absence of a usable gastrointestinal tract intravenous nutrition (TPN) can be used. A sterile dedicated central line, with a bacterial filter, is needed, as infection is an ever-present concern. The TPN bag is shielded from the light in a red bag, to prevent the degradation of water soluble vitamins. The sterile preparation of a pre-mixed recipe has simplified the process.

LEAKAGE OF TPN

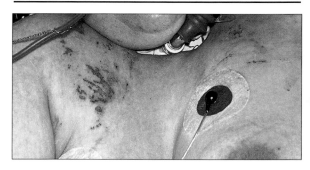

Fig. 79 This subclavian line produced swelling and excoriation of the skin. A hole had been made in the catheter during insertion.

PANCREATITIS

ACUTE PANCREATITIS: GREY TURNER'S SIGN AND CULLEN'S SIGN

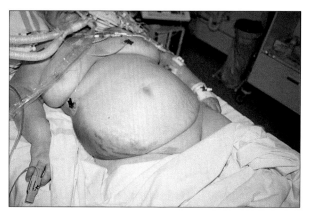

Fig. 80 Bruising of the flank (Grey Turner's sign) shows desperate disease. Pancreatitis is a very deceptive illness. There may be little in the way of clinical signs despite unrelenting disease. The serum amylase may be transiently increased during the acute illness, but normal in the chronic situation. Symptoms include harsh pain often relieved by sitting forward, vomiting and dehydration. Cullen's sign (bruising around the umbilicus) is visible in this patient as well.

NECROTISING PANCREATITIS

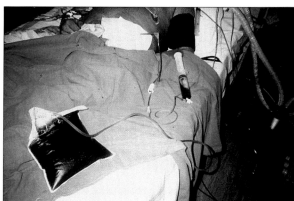

Fig. 81 Typical 'prune juice' obtained after peritoneal lavage in acute necrotising pancreatitis. The amylase was 22,000 units/l on this specimen. There is no evidence that this procedure alters the bad prognosis in these patients.

CT SCAN OF PANCREAS

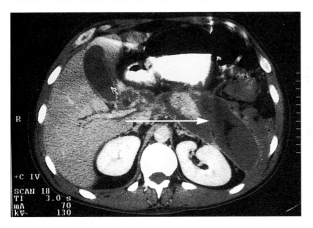

Fig. 82 A massive pancreatic abscess (arrow) with destruction of the tail of the pancreas. Aspiration by a fine needle sample at this time grew *Escherichia coli*. A CT scan is a useful procedure after the acute attack, to identify a pseudocyst, phlegmon or abscess. The principle causes of pancreatitis are alcohol abuse and gallstones, and to a lesser extent trauma, drugs, and infections.

PANCREATITIS: DIC

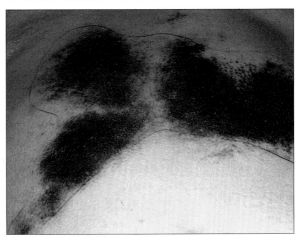

Fig. 83 A combination of DIC (shown here), ARDS and renal failure are poor prognostic signs seen in necrotising pancreatitis. A mortality of at least 60% can be expected.

LIVER DISEASE

ASCITES

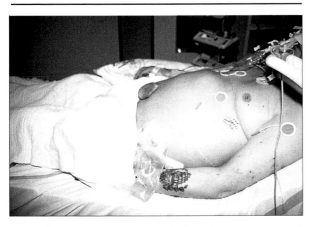

Fig. 84 This patient collapsed after decompression of his tense ascites. He also has an umbilical hernia. The drainage site continues to leak yellow ascitic fluid (seen at bottom of the picture). A sample of ascitic fluid should always be sent for culture. Free fluid in the abdomen can cause excruciating pain, compromise respiration (see **Fig. 190**, p. 56) and become infected.

HEPATOSPLENOMEGALY

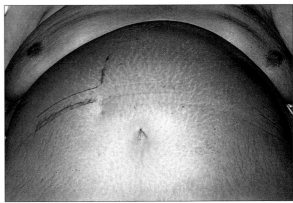

Fig. 85 Enormous enlargement of the liver (marked) with a palpable spleen plus ascites was found on palpation in this patient needing ventilatory support. The liver may be pushed down if large tidal volumes or high levels of PEEP are used. This does not affect the spleen.

CAPUT MEDUSA

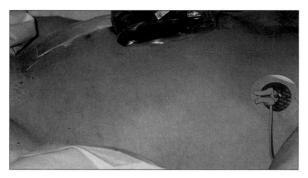

Fig. 86 The presence of portal hypertension can lead to distension of collateral veins, in this case over the abdominal wall. It was secondary to a ruptured liver.

LIVER PALM

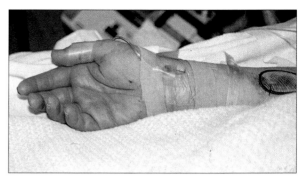

Fig. 87 In contrast to the jaundiced forearm the palm becomes red because of a hyperdynamic circulation and vasodilation.

LIVER FLAP

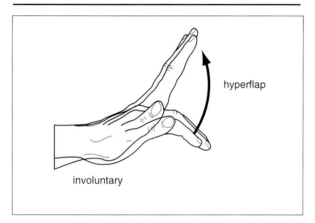

hyperflap

involuntary

Fig. 88 An irregular flap (so-called after the wings of a bird in flight) occurs in liver disease.

DUPUYTREN'S CONTRACTURE

Fig. 89 This is a flexion deformity of the ring and/or little finger cause by thickening of the palmar fascia. The thickened fascia can be felt; it is often bilateral and is associated with alcoholic cirrhosis. This patient also has a liver palm.

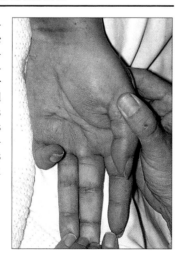

SPIDER NAEVI

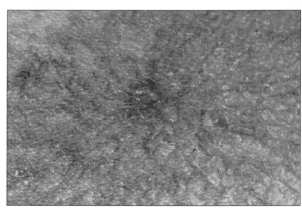

Fig. 90 A large spider naevus. The presence of multiple spider naevi over the face, chest and upper arms is suggestive of liver disease.

GYNAECOMASTIA

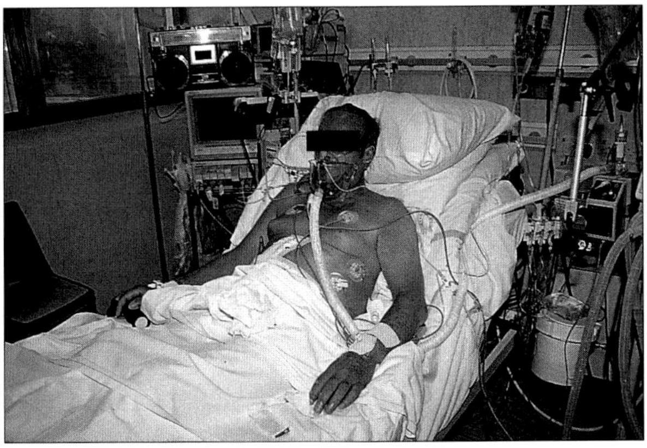

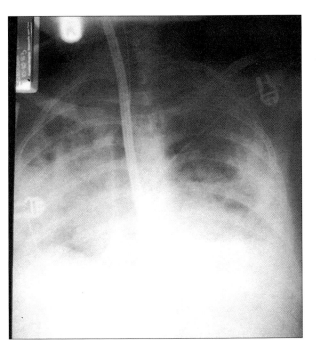

Fig. 91 Caused by oestrogen accumulation. This man has chronic liver disease and had a transplant 24 hours before this picture was taken.

HAEMATEMESIS: SENSTRAKEN-BLAKEMORE TUBE

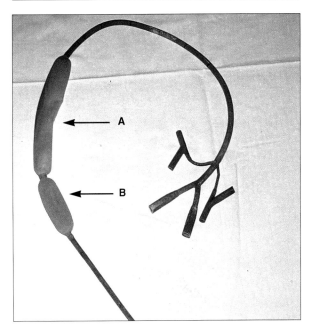

Fig. 92 The Senstraken-Blakemore tube is used to compress bleeding oesophageal varices. It is passed through the nose (first having corrected any clotting defect) or the mouth and positioned with the lower gastric balloon (B, arrow) in the stomach and the longer oesophageal balloon (A, arrow) along the length of the oesophagus.

CHEST RADIOGRAPH OF POSITION OF SENSTRAKEN-BLAKEMORE TUBE; ASPIRATION OF BLOOD

Fig. 93 The size and pointed tip of the tube can cause damage on insertion and a radiograph should be taken after placement as the tube has a habit of curling in the oesophagus. This is a simple method of compression of varices that works with 90% of patients. The chest radiograph also shows pulmonary aspiration of blood has occurred.

BLEEDING VARICES: RADIOLOGICAL INTERVENTION

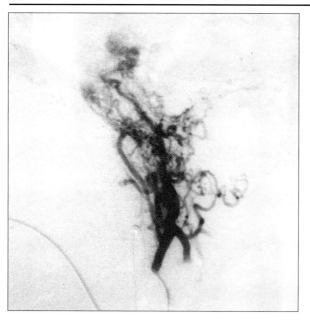 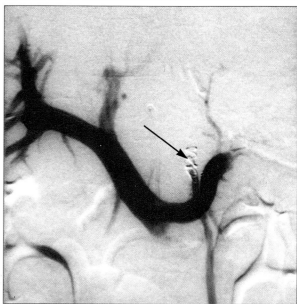

Figs 94 and **95** Failure of medical treatment may need radiological intervention. Here a cluster of varices (**94**, left) have been successfully ablated with a metal coil inserted at their origin (arrow, **95**, right).

GASTROINTESTINAL BLEEDING

HAEMATEMESIS: COFFEE GROUNDS

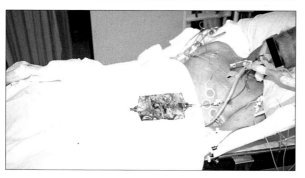

Fig. 96 This patient has 'coffee ground' aspirates draining up the nasogastric tube. Upper gastro-intestinal bleeding is a feature of severe illness. The 'coffee grounds' show that the blood is old and continuing bleeding is unlikely when they occur.

HAEMATEMESIS: ACUTE BLEEDING

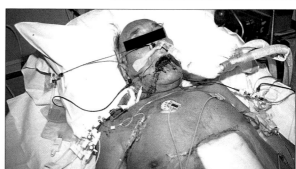

Fig. 97 This patient has started to vomit large amounts of fresh red blood. Bleeding is now occurring.

HAEMATEMESIS: BLOOD LOSS

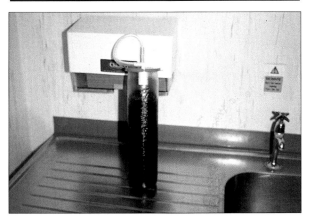

Fig. 98 The patient lost this amount of blood in four hours. Endoscopy revealed a severe oesophagitis.

STRESS ULCERS

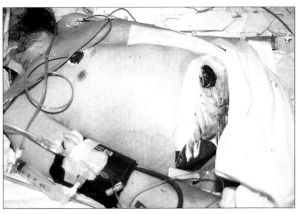

Fig. 99 Stress ulcers occur in burns, sepsis, renal and hepatic failure and head injuries despite the use of drugs such as sucralfate and ranitidine to prevent them.

ENDOSCOPY OF ULCER

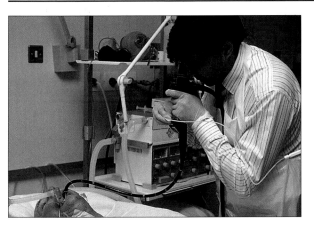 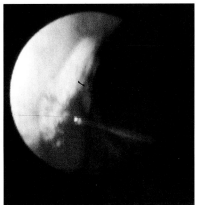

Figs 100 and **101** Persistent bleeding requires an endoscopy to diagnose the cause (**100**, left). Here the source is obvious (**101**, right).

ANGIOGRAPHY OF BLEEDING VESSEL

Fig. 102 Radiological help can demonstrate the bleeding site. Here a selective injection of the left gastric artery reveals the spurting ulcer. This can then be embolised on the spot without recourse to surgery, saving the patient an operation.

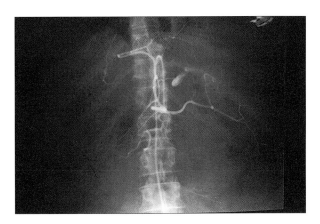

RUPTURED OESOPHAGUS

Figs 103 and **104** The chest radiograph (**103,** left) shows two features of a ruptured oesophagus, namely a pneumothorax and fluid collection (shown also in diagram, **104,** right). The patient wrenched her shoulder getting out of a train, felt a sharp pain in her chest but did not seek medical help until she developed respiratory failure secondary to an empyema a week later.

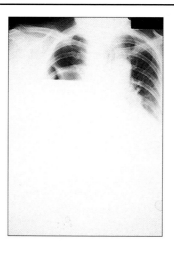
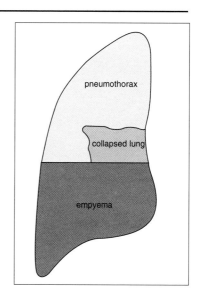

RENAL FAILURE

Acute renal failure is a serious complication. Causes include hypotension and ischaemia; pancreatitis; diarrhoea; crush injury; rhabdomyolysis; grave sepsis; pregnancy; drugs (notably antibiotics such as gentamicin) and radiographic dyes. Although oliguria is a predominant feature, 20% of cases present as polyuria.

RENAL BIOPSY

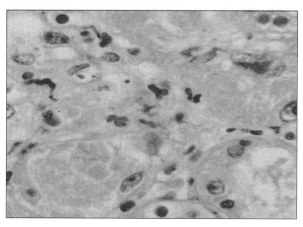

Fig. 105 The biopsy, undertaken with ultrasound guided control, shows the typical features of acute tubular necrosis. Dilated dead and degenerating tubules are filled with debris, separated by oedema fluid.

ULTRASOUND OF KIDNEY

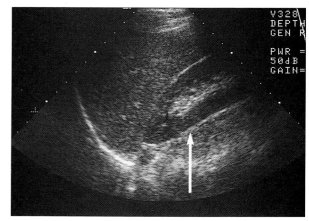

Fig. 106 Ultrasound is an important investigation giving useful information about the renal system. If it is normal and there is no clear cause for the renal failure (such as hypotension) then a renal biopsy may be needed.

CONJUNCTIVAL OEDEMA

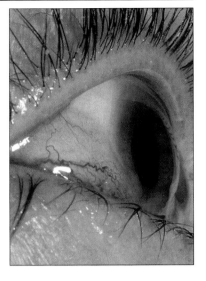

Fig. 107 Conjunctival oedema with facial puffiness and more generalised oedema is a feature of acute renal failure.

RENAL INFARCT

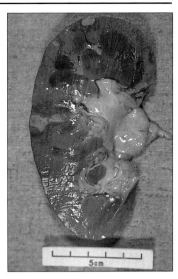

Fig. 108 This kidney shows discrete pale infarcted lesions. If all the cortex is involved the kidney cannot recover.

PERITONEAL DIALYSIS

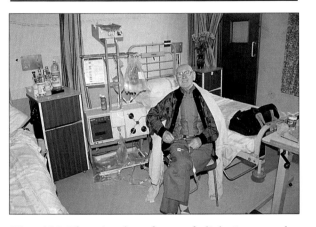

Fig. 109 The simplest form of dialysis uses the peritoneal cavity. The dialysis fluid is put into the abdominal cavity, left there for a while then drained out. Urea, potassium and other substances 'dialyse' into this fluid. Because large amounts of fluid are used, patients suffer from cold even if the fluids are warmed.

PERITONEAL DIALYSIS: FLUID BALANCE

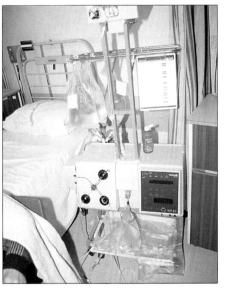

Fig. 110 The large fluid input/output used during peritoneal dialysis is greatly aided by automatic balances. Peritoneal dialysis can be extremely effective but may not be a practical proposition in the critically ill, because of previous abdominal surgery and interference with breathing.

HAEMODIALYSIS

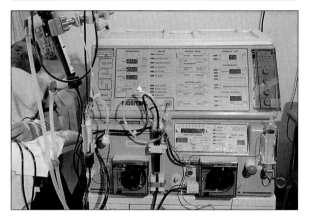

Fig. 111 Haemodialysis is a difficult undertaking in acute illness, because of the haemodynamic instability it causes. All forms of haemodialysis need an extracorporeal circuit, which necessitates anticoagulation to prevent blood clotting. Heparin can be used, but if there is a risk of bleeding prostacyclin can be used instead. Various columns can be used to remove fluids or enable some drugs to be cleared.

HAEMODIALYSIS: VASCULAR ACCESS

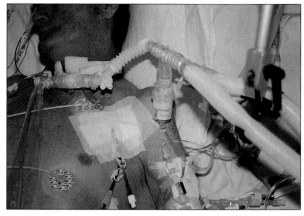

Fig. 112 There are two ways to provide access for haemodialysis. A subclavian or femoral vein dialysis catheter can be inserted as a temporary solution, as shown here. They are likely to become clotted or infected if used for long periods, but they do provide the most suitable means of access in critically ill patients. For long-term dialysis an arterio-venous fistula in the arm or leg is constructed.

HAEMOFILTRATION

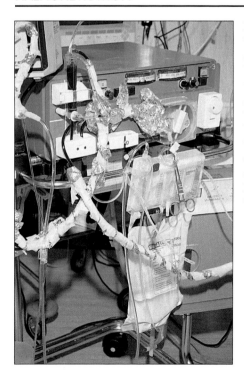

Fig. 113 This is an example of continuous veno-venous haemofiltration and dialysis. This method uses a venous access line and the blood is pumped through a filter. The ultrafiltrate collected in the bag is yellow (as seen in the photograph), its colour caused by the excretion of urokines. Dialysis fluid can also be pumped around the filter, which increases the clearance of toxins. This is an extremely efficient system that does not usually cause the collapse of the patient and runs continuously. Dehydration is easy to achieve. Silver foil is used to prevent heat loss.

DRUG REACTIONS

PHLEBITIS OF THE LEG

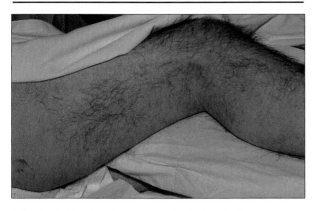

Fig. 114 The leg is not an ideal site for intravenous infusions. This reaction along the length of the vein occurred after intravenous antibiotics. The use of leg veins may also predispose to the development of a deep vein thrombosis.

GENERALISED ALLERGIC RASH

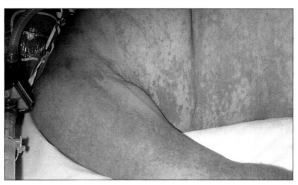

Fig. 115 It can be difficult to decide which drug or infusion is the culprit. Antibiotics remain the most common cause.

VASCULITIS

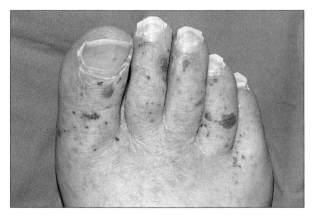

Fig. 116 A vasculitic rash secondary to drug administration.

BILATERAL GANGRENE CAUSED BY VASCULITIS

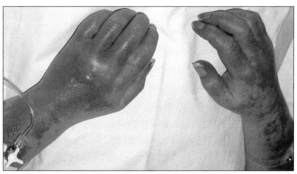

Fig. 117 This extreme reaction to diazide resulted in a severe vasculitis.

URTICARIA/ANAPHYLACTIC REACTION

Fig. 118 'Nettle rash' over the body is a common and milder presentation of an allergic reaction. Generalised oedema with cardiovascular collapse occurs in acute anaphylactic reactions.

SYSTEMIC VASCULITIS CAUSED BY DRUGS

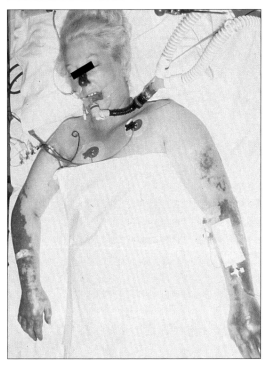

Fig. 119 Generalised vasculitis of all limbs including the nose.

STEVENS-JOHNSON (LYELL'S) SYNDROME

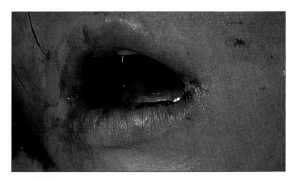

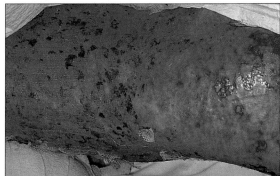

Figs 120 and **121** The syndrome is characterised by exfoliation with unpleasant involvement of mucous membranes secondary to drug administration (**120**, upper). It is thankfully quite rare. **Fig. 121** (lower) shows extensive skin loss and blistering over the torso.

TRAUMA

Trauma is the leading cause of death in young people. The major recent advances in the care of this demanding group have been the provision of expert site-of-injury resuscitation by trained paramedics; the training of hospital staff in resuscitation protocols (e.g. ATLS) and the creation of trauma centres and ICUs where skilled nursing can support the recovery stage.

There are different mechanisms of injury, such as crush (car accident or fall) and penetrating (stabbing or gunshot wound) injuries. The type of injury determines the nature of the underlying damage and in general terms the greater the speed of injury occurs the more extensive the damage.

OXYGEN AND AIRWAY

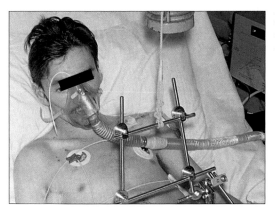

Fig. 122 The first requirement is a clear airway and adequate oxygenation.

'CHARLIES' VEIN

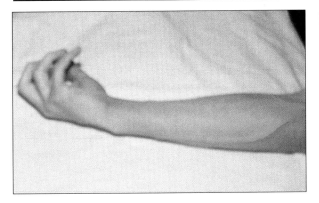

Fig. 123 Resuscitation needs good intravenous access. The anastomotic veins at the side of the forearm are often overlooked and provide excellent large entry sites. The mnemonic 'CHARLIES' (**C**hoose **H**is **A**rm **R**ight and **L**eft w**I**th **E**a**S**e) can be helpful in remembering this fact.

CHEST DRAIN

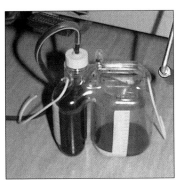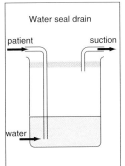

Figs 125 and **126** Life-threatening conditions such a pneumothorax or haemothorax must be treated with a chest drain (**125**, left). A large number of deaths after trauma are caused by thoracic injuries. The water seal drain shown in the diagram (**126**, right) works as a one-way valve by passing any air that escapes through a water trap. If a large leak occurs, two drains in series need to be used. Low pressure suction helps re-expand the lung.

FRACTURED RIBS

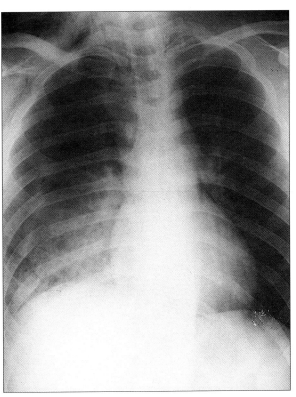

Fig. 124 There are fractures down the entire right side of this man's chest. Surgical emphysema of the neck is also seen, and he has aspirated vomit into his right lung.

FLAIL CHEST/REGIONAL ANALGESIA

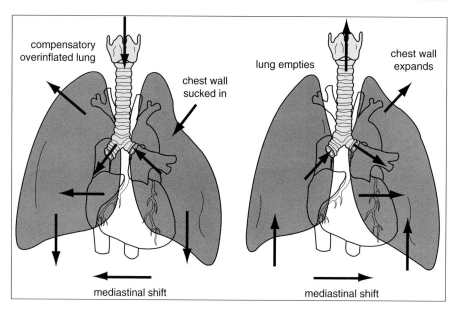

Fig. 127 This diagram shows the mechanism of respiratory failure in the presence of a flail segment. Mechanical ventilation is sometimes needed to stabilise the situation. Good analgesia is important and regional blockade (epidural or intercostal blocks) ideal.

Table 4 Relationship of zone of rib fracture and associated injuries

Zone	Site	Associated injury
A	ribs 1–4 clavicle	major vessels ruptured bronchus/trachea brachial plexus
B	ribs 5–9	flail chest lung contusion
C	ribs 10–12	laceration to liver/spleen kidney damage ruptured diaphragm

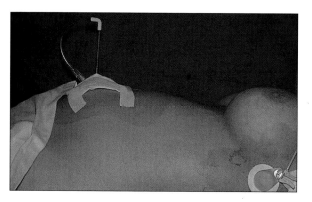

'MICHELIN WOMAN'

Fig. 128 Generalised surgical emphysema. Always think of a ruptured trachea or bronchus when this is so marked. In this patient air has also tracked between the crus of the diaphragm, distending the abdomen. This interfered with artificial ventilation and was relieved with a peritoneal dialysis catheter, as shown.

STERNAL INJURY

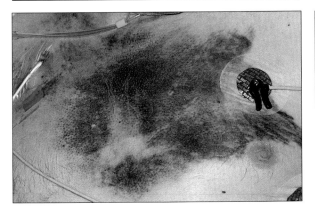

Fig. 129 Such a violent blow to the chest can lead to shearing forces tearing mobile organs, such as the heart, from the adjacent arteries or rupture the aorta; abdominal organs can suffer a similar fate.

STERNAL INJURY: SEAT BELT INJURY

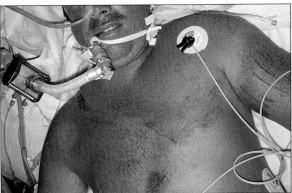

Fig. 130 The line of the seat belt is visible here. Crush injuries can also occur, compressing the sternum against the spine and involving the liver, spleen and pancreas. There may be few external signs. Myocardial infarction is possible in this type of injury.

GUNSHOT WOUNDS TO CHEST

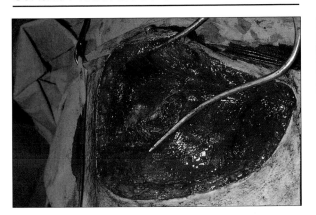

Fig. 131 High-velocity bullets cause great damage to the body, and result in cavitation of surrounding tissue. Changes in direction and fragmentation lead to complex and surprising injuries. Stabbing tends to cause more localised damage.

CHEST RADIOGRAPH OF TRAUMATIC LUNG PSEUDOCYSTS AND LEFT PNEUMOTHORAX

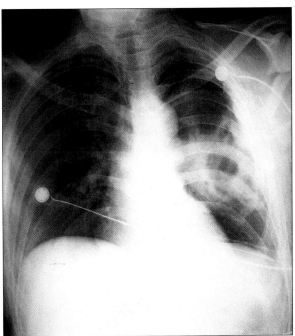

Fig. 132 Caused by injury in a helicopter crash.

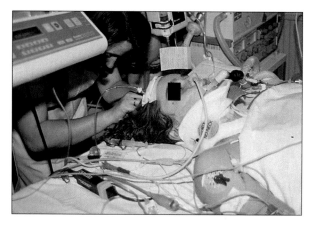

HEAD INJURY

Fig. 133 This girl fell off her horse six hours previously and became unconscious. She underwent a CT scan of the head which showed cerebral oedema but no haemorrhage. Her lungs are being ventilated mechanically to lower her intracranial pressure (see **Fig. 156**, p. 45). A neck-brace has been put on whilst her condition is being stabilised and in case she has a cervical injury.

NECK TRACTION

Figs 134 and **135** This patient has a fractured cervical spine; he has been stabilised in neck traction.

Neck injuries should be considered from the moment a trauma victim is first seen.

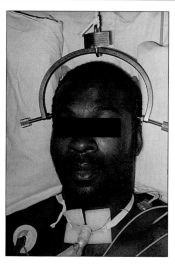
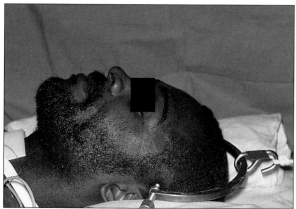

EMPYEMA FOLLOWING STAB WOUND TO CHEST

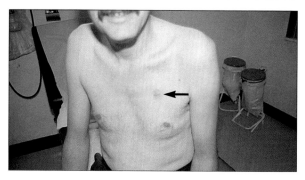
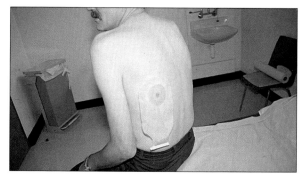

Figs 136 and **137** A domestic argument led to a carving knife being stabbed into this man's chest (site of wound indicated by arrow). This led to an empyema that had to be surgically drained.

MULTIPLE INJURIES

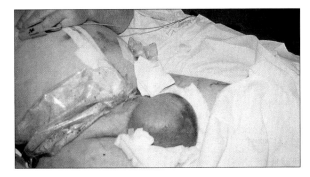

Fig. 138 Extensive injuries caused by a motor-cycle accident. Aluminium foil is wrapped around the body to retain body heat. Rapid surgery was required to control haemorrhage and over 60 units of blood were needed during the operation. Peritoneal lavage had shown a grossly bloodstained specimen. A ruptured spleen was removed. Abdominal injuries may be overlooked when such extensive limb injuries occur.

Haemorrhage and head injury are the immediate causes of death after trauma.

SCROTAL HAEMATOMA

Fig. 139 Significant bleeding in the abdomen can result in blood tracking down to the genitalia and gross swelling.

INTRAVENOUS PYELOGRAM (IVP) AFTER TRAUMA

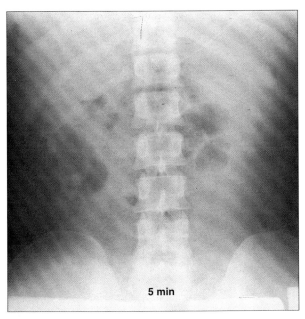

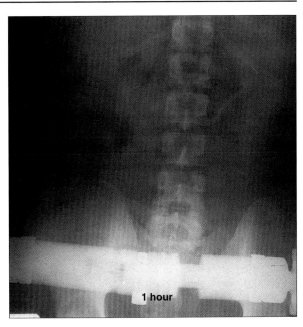

Figs 140 and **141** This man was trapped in a car for some hours before arrival in hospital, having suffered a severe crush injury. He underwent an IVP which shows at 5 minutes (**140,** left) and 1 hour (**141,** right) a total absence of renal function. He required urgent dialysis because of a rapidly increasing potassium level.

WARM AIR BLOWER

Fig. 142 A simple but very effective warm air blower is used to arrest decline in core temperature, but also to return it to normal. Trauma patients can be trapped for hours and may be partially clad in Casualty and remain so in the operating theatre. Rewarming is needed to prevent hypothermia. Another method is to use a fluidised bed (see **Fig. 68**, p. 23).

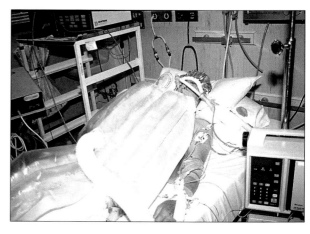

PATIENT-CONTROLLED ANALGESIA (PCA)

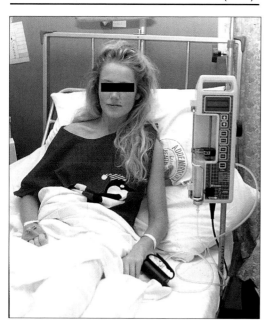

Fig. 143 Intravenous morphine administered by the patient to him or herself results in perfect pain control. An antiemetic should be always given as well.

PAIN ASSESSMENT CHART

OPIOID PCA / INFUSION CHART

ACUTE PAIN SERVICE

Patient Details
Name: Date: ....
Hospital No: Operation: ....
Age: Anaesthetist: ....
Sex: Ward: ....ITU/Recovery.....................
ASA I II III IV V Emergency/Elective   Regional Technique: Epidural   SAB
                                                                      Caudal   Sciatic
Drug Treatment i.e. Opioids, Antiemetics   Femoral   Brachial
Pre-Op: Infiltration
                                                                      Ihioinguinal
Intra-Op: Other   ....
Post-Op: Indication: Operative / Medical Problem

STANDING ORDERS

Morphine   1mg/ml*
Pethidine   10mg/ml*   MADE UP TO A VOLUME OF 50 MLS
                                                NORMAL SALINE
Antiemetic   ....   *PLEASE DELETE AS APPROPRIATE
LOADING/BOLUS DOSES (Morphine/Pethidine*)   ....mg, repeat after 10 minutes if pain
                                                control is not adequate. Ensure Loading doses
                                                are documented in the Loading\Bolus Given Box.

                          SIGNATURE ....

SETTINGS

DATE	DRUG	PCA DOSE	LOCKOUT	4 HRLY LIMIT	BACKGROUND	SIGNATURE
	MORPHINE	1 MG	5 MIN			

LOADING/BOLUS GIVEN

DATE/TIME	DOSE	SIGNATURE	DATE/TIME	DOSE	SIGNATURE

REFILLS

DATE	TIME	AMOUNT DISCARD	SIGNATURE	DATE	TIME	AMOUNT DISCARD	SIGNATURE

Fig. 144 A pain assessment chart is needed to supervise management of pain.

EPIDURAL INFUSION

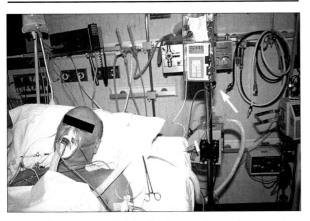

Fig. 145 Regional blockade is the other main method of pain control. This is usually a combination of analgesia and local anaesthetic, controlled again by a PCA (see **Fig. 143**, p. 42), or a continuous infusion machine (indicated by arrow) and managed with a pain assessment chart similar to the one shown in **Fig. 144**, p. 42.

KETAMINE

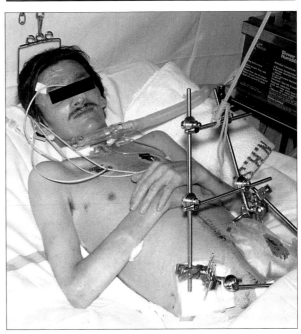

Fig. 146 This 19-year-old man was involved in a road-traffic accident. He landed on the gearstick of the car he was driving, suffering a pelvic fracture and a gaping perineal laceration. This required daily packing. Pain control was eventually achieved by an intravenous ketamine infusion.

NEUROLOGY

OVERDOSE

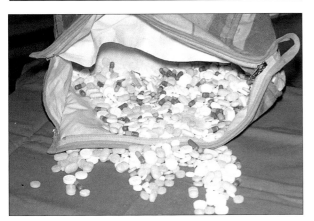

Fig. 147 There are often few clinical signs. Until proved otherwise the primary cause of coma in an adult under 40 years is an overdose. All patients need to have an intact airway, adequate oxygenation, be nursed in a lateral position and if the gag reflex is poor, to be protected from aspiration by a nasogastric tube and a tracheal tube. Blood sugar should be routinely measured to exclude hypoglycaemia.

METABOLIC AND MORPHINE-INDUCED COMA

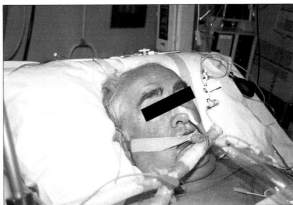

Fig. 148 This man had received a morphine infusion for five days despite being unconscious and in acute renal failure. The metabolite of morphine, morphine-6-glucuronide, is excreted by the kidney. He woke up when he started to pass urine.

The presence of renal or hepatic failure, often in combination with sedatives and analgesics in the ICU, can make the assessment of cerebral function a difficult task.

NORMAL CT OF BRAIN IN METABOLIC COMA

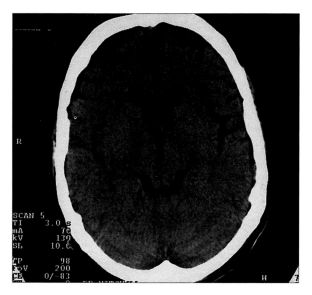

Fig. 149 This 43-year-old patient with renal failure suffered a septic episode and had some features of upper motor changes in the arms. There was no papilloedema. A lumbar puncture revealed slight xanthrochromia suggesting a previous haemorrhage. The CT scan is entirely normal. He recovered slowly over a period of seven days. The cause of his coma was never established but probably involved a general metabolic derangement and drug intoxication.

DECEREBRATE POSTURE

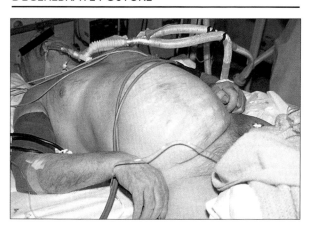

Fig. 151 A decerebrate posture following a cardiac arrest.

POSTURES

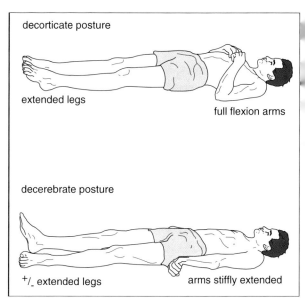

decorticate posture

extended legs

full flexion arms

decerebrate posture

+/_ extended legs

arms stiffly extended

Fig. 150 The body may respond with some characteristic movements in severe brain damage.

NEUROTOXIC REACTION

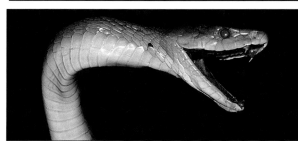

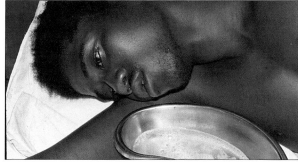

Figs 152 and **153** The bite of the black mamba (**152**, top) leads to ptosis with inability to swallow with hypersalivation (**153**, lower).

Table 5: Glasgow Coma Scale (GCS)

Best verbal response		Best motor response		Eyes open	
Orientated	5	Obeys commands	6	Spontaneously	4
Confused	4	Localises to pain	5	to command	3
Inappropriate words	3	Withdraws to pain	4	To pain	2
Incomprehensible sounds	2	Flexion to pain	3	None	0
None	1	Extension to pain	2		
		None	0		

The level of coma can be assessed and followed using the Glasgow Coma Scale (GCS).

PAPILLOEDEMA

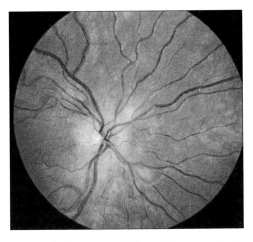

Fig. 154 The normal sharp disc margin has become blurred. This is one of the few clinical signs that indicate raised ICP (intracranial pressure). The majority of head injuries will have raised ICP.

PRESSURE/VOLUME RELATIONSHIP IN ICP

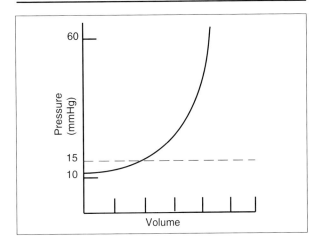

Fig. 155 The normal ICP is below 15 mmHg. The relationship between volume and pressure shows little increase in pressure at first despite an increasing brain size. Compensatory shifts of CSF and blood maintain a normal ICP, but are limited. The curve then becomes a dangerously steep incline over 15 mmHg.

MEASUREMENT OF ICP

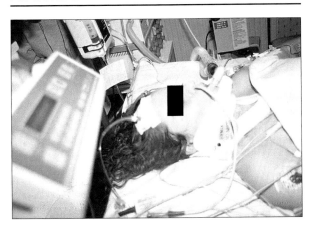

Fig. 156 This patient with a head injury has had a subarachnoid bolt inserted to monitor intracranial pressure continuously. The normal cerebral perfusion pressure (i.e. the difference between mean arterial pressure and ICP) is >60mm Hg. Autoregulation ceases below 40 mmHg.

CT SCAN: CEREBRAL OEDEMA

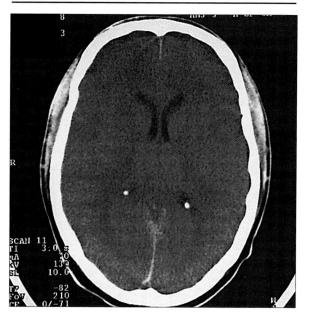

Fig. 157 Compared to the normal CT (see **Fig. 149**, p. 44) there is a total loss of cerebral architecture. This patient is brain-dead secondary to cerebral oedema.

TESTS FOR BRAIN DEATH

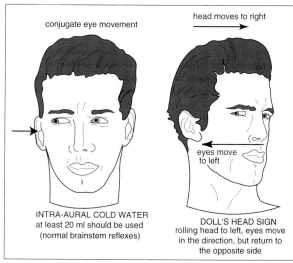

Fig. 158 These include:
A. fixed, dilated pupils
B. absent corneal reflex
C. no eye movement on installation of intra-aural cold water
D. no response on using doll's head manoeuvre
E. no cranial nerve response
F. no gag reflex
G. no spontaneous respiration after discontinuation of ventilation with $PaCO_2$ >6.7 kPa – check blood gases.

CT SCAN OF SUBARACHNOID HAEMORRHAGE

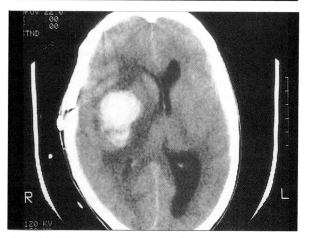

Fig. 159 The diagnosis is usually obvious. A very sharp headache is reported, with vomiting and often a transient loss of consciousness. The CSF is grossly blood-stained. A 'berry' aneurysm of the Circle of Willis is the usual cause, as shown here.

CEREBRAL ANGIOGRAM

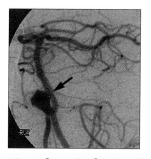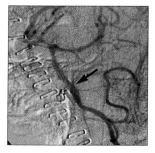

Figs 160 and **161** The diagnosis of aneurysm (arrow, **160**, left) is confirmed by angiography. The treatment is surgical 'clipping' (arrow, **161**, right).

CT: HEAD INJURY

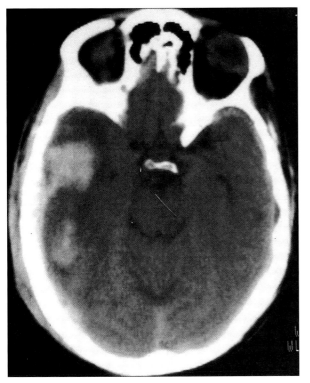

Fig. 162 This scan shows cerebral contusion with intracerebral haemorrhage. Early CT scanning of a head injury ensures that haematomas, which can be treated surgically, are not missed.

CHRONIC SUBDURAL HAEMATOMA

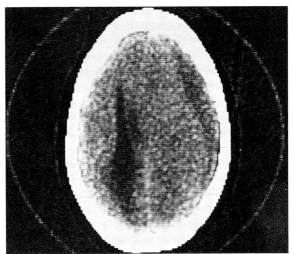

Fig. 163 Non-specific neurological signs can occur in the presence of subdural haematoma. Trivial trauma can sometimes cause a subdural haematoma in the elderly, resulting in death if not diagnosed.

SUBCONJUCTIVAL HAEMORRHAGE

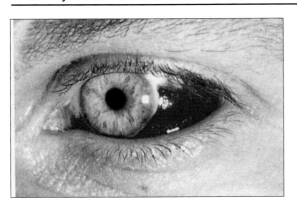

Fig. 164 A red eye resulting from a blow to the face.

CEREBRAL FUNCTION MONITOR: STATUS EPILEPTICUS/THIOPENTONE INFUSION

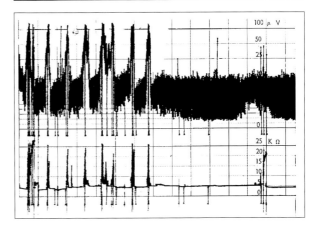

Fig. 165 Recurrent epileptic fits were diagnosed on this cerebral function monitor trace. Giving sufficient anticonvulsants to stop this may cause respiratory depression. Mechanical ventilation overcomes this concern. In this case a thiopentone infusion was used after repeated boluses of diazepam had failed, with a dramatic effect.

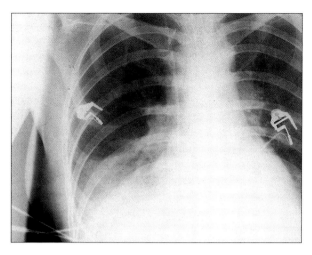

BULBAR PALSY: ASPIRATION

Fig. 166 This 22-year-old secretary presented with swallowing problems resulting in pulmonary aspiration of stomach contents. Her blood gases (see **Tables 6** and **7** below) also deteriorated to a stage where ventilation was required (note the increased $PaCO_2$, **Table 7**). A biopsy revealed dermatomyositis. Recovery was slow and required eight weeks of ventilatory support but she improved and was discharged. She still cannot coordinate her swallowing properly at eight months.

Table 6 Blood gases over 48 hours (1)

Temperature	36.5°C
F_IO_2	0.30
Measured at	37.0°C
pH	7.387
$PaCO_2$	6.57 kPa
PaO_2	12.0 kPa

Table 7 Blood gases over 48 hours (2)

F_IO2	0.30
Measured at	37.0°C
pH	7.316
$PaCO_2$	8.57 kPa
PaO_2	10.6 kPa

MYASTHENIA GRAVIS

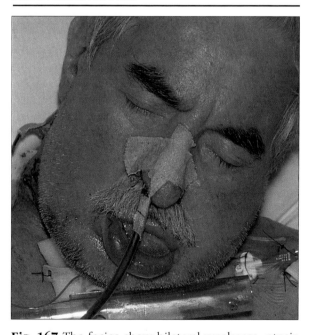

Fig. 167 The facies show bilateral weakness, ptosis and a characteristic 'snarl'. Myasthenia can also present as a bulbar palsy. The condition is characterised by rapid fatigue on exertion. Patients present to the ICU with swallowing and respiratory difficulties.

GUILLAIN-BARRÉ SYNDROME: FACIES

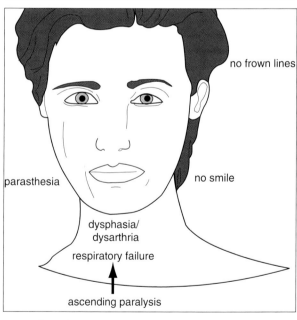

Fig. 168 Bilateral flaccid limb weakness often spreads to affect facial muscles, giving this bland appearance. Early treatment with plasmaphoresis can limit the severity of the disease and speed recovery. The disease is self-limiting: recovery can take months.

MYOPATHY

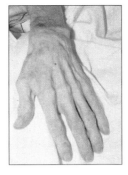

Fig. 169 This 53-year-old man's hand shows marked wasting. He was still unable to stand four months after a liver transplant. An electromyogram confirmed a distal myopathy. This condition has been underdiagnosed in the ICU, especially after protracted illness. The use of muscle relaxants and steroids make it worse.

GROSS WASTING DUE TO INACTIVITY

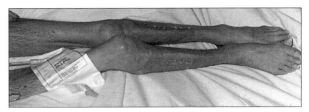

Fig. 170 The weakness here is because of catabolism in a critically ill patient who has been bedridden for three months. There is no neuromuscular disorder.

TRANSPORT OF CRITICALLY ILL PATIENTS

TRANSFER BY RAIL

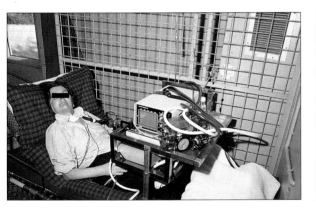

Fig. 171 Long-term patients travel well. There are good mobile monitoring and ventilation units available. This patient was transferred from Edinburgh to London by train.

TRANSFER BY ROAD

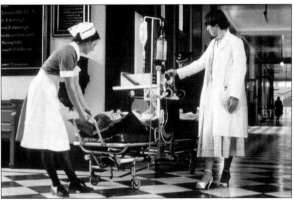

Fig. 172 The most usual mode of transfer is by road. Paramedic ambulances are now available, and a doctor must accompany the patient.

TRANSFER BY AIR

Fig. 173 Repatriation can occur across vast distances if properly organised.

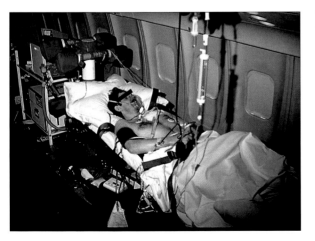

SHOCK

Shock is a condition in which inadequate tissue perfusion leads to progressive organ dysfunction. This is often as a result of a low cardiac output, but high output situations exist, e.g. sepsis. Unless the situation can be arrested, irreversible organ failure and death will occur. Priorities include stabilising the cardiorespiratory systems by mechanical ventilation if necessary to maintain an SpO_2 >90%, a MAP over 70 mmHg and a urine output of 1 ml/kg per hour. A mortality of 70% is reported in most centres.

POOR PERFUSION OF THE LIMBS

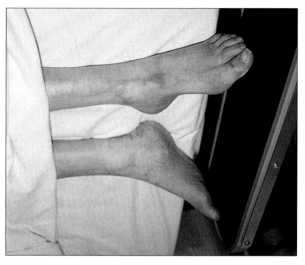

Fig. 174 A cold, poorly perfused periphery is the classical presentation of shock. Hypotension and a tachycardia accompany this situation.

PAIN: ACUTE PERFORATION OF ABDOMINAL VISCUS

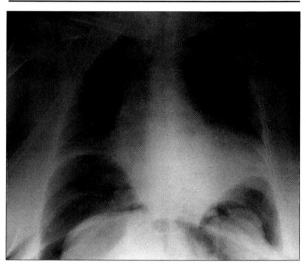

Fig. 175 Air is present under both diaphragms. Relief of pain is an immediate priority, often neglected, in the management of shock.

Table 8: Causes of shock

Low cardiac output	examples: Hypovolaemia	examples: trauma, burns, GI losses, haemorrhage
	Cardiogenic shock	examples: MI, arrythmia
High output state	examples: Sepsis	
	Liver failure	
Obstructive	examples: Pneumothorax	
	Cardiac tamponade	
	CPAP	
Other	Vagal	
	Anaphylaxis	
	Neurological	

A wide variety of diseases can result in shock.

RADIOGRAPH OF GUNSHOT WOUNDS TO ABDOMEN

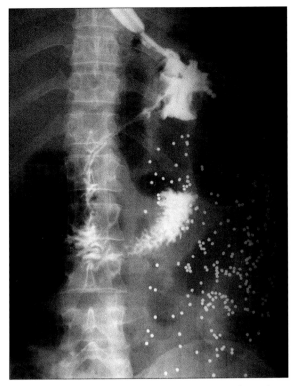

Fig. 176 This extensive injury produced a combination of hypovolaemic, septic and neurological induced shock.

HYPOVOLAEMIC SHOCK: LEAKING AORTIC ANEURYSM

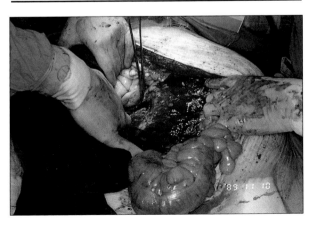

Fig. 178 The surgeon has clamped the neck of the leaking aorta. There is extensive bleeding. Aggressive fluid replacement is always indicated. At least two large bore intravenous lines are needed. Blood loss can exceed 20 units of blood.

CT OF GUNSHOT WOUNDS TO ABDOMEN

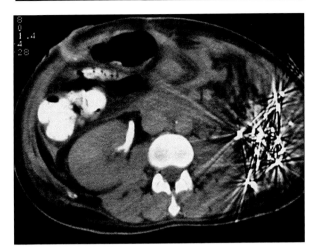

Fig. 177 Some visual idea of the extensive damage produced by bullet wounds can be gained from looking at this CT of an abdomen injured by gunshot wounds.

CARDIOGENIC SHOCK

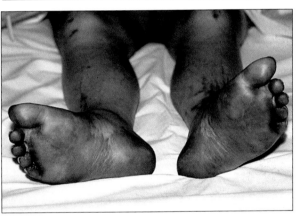

Fig. 179 Cyanosed feet indicating a low output state secondary to myocardial infarction. Monitoring with an arterial line and pulmonary artery catheter (PAC) permits constant and careful supervision of such cases. Offloading the heart with nitrates is often beneficial. An echocardiogram is essential in the presence of a persistent shocked state, to exclude a ruptured valve, septal defect or surgically correctable lesion.

ECG OF MYOCARDIAL INFARCT

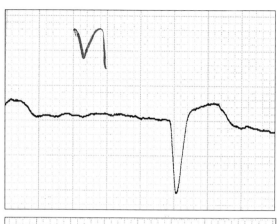

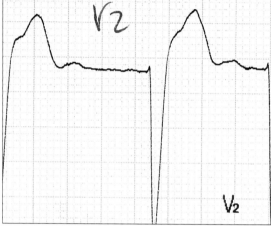

Fig. 180 The classical deep Q wave and raised ST segment of an acute myocardial infarct.

SEPTIC SHOCK

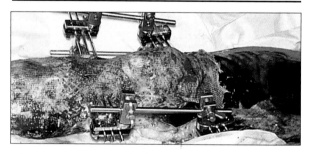

Fig. 182 A crushed, burned and septic leg. A farmworker kicked a bale of hay into a bailing machine and his leg was trapped inside.

Septic shock, unlike the other types discussed, is characterised by a high cardiac output (see **Table 2** and **Table 3**, p. 16). The hypotension that occurs is due to vasodilation.

OBSTRUCTIVE SHOCK: PULMONARY EMBOLISM

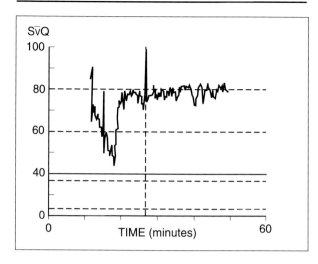

Fig. 181 This substantial decrease in venous oxygen tension occurred due to a pulmonary embolism (see Chapter 4, Cardiology).

LOW OUTPUT STATE: CARDIAC OUTPUT MEASUREMENT

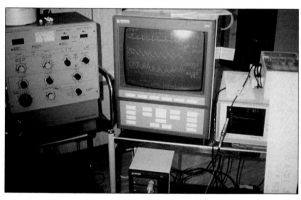

Fig. 183 Sophisticated monitoring equipment is needed to understand the clinical process. Two classes of drugs are used in shock: vasopressors and vasodilators. They have their limitations. To evaluate their actions and follow the progress of ill patients an aggressive policy is required if patients are to survive.

Table 9 Management of a low cardiac output state after myocardial infarct

The findings were:	Measured	Normal range
1. A low cardiac index {cardiac output/surface area}	1.45	2.8–3.6 l/min/m^2
2. A normal systemic vascular resistance (SVRI)	1721	>1760–2600 dyne/sec/cm^{-5}
3. A very low mean arterial pressure (MAP)	51	>70 mmHg
4. A normal wedge pressure (PCWP)	14	6–12 mmHg
5. Very poor oxygen delivery and consumption	330/140	520–720/100–180 ml/min/m^2

The first step is restoration of mean arterial pressure (MAP) and cardiac output using inotropes to ensure adequate coronary artery blood flow. In view of the adequate filling pressures and normal systemic resistance, dobutamine was given. The patient is being mechanically ventilated to ensure good oxygenation. The haemoglobin was acceptable so urgent blood transfusion was not needed, but it is likely that the vasodilation produced will need colloid support.

Table 10 Improved cardiac output after treatment

Input values				
Ht	163 cm	64 in		
Wt	60 kg	133 lb		
MAP	90 mmHg	PaO$_2$	9	kPa
CVP	10 mmHg	SaO$_2$	99	%
MPA	31 mmHg	S$\overline{v}$O$_2$	79	%
PCWP	24 mmHg	Hb	9.8	g/dl

Calculated values			
AVG CO	5.14	CaO$_2$ (99)	13.2
AVG CI	3.12	C$\overline{v}$O$_2$ (79)	10.5
BSA	1.65	$\dot{D}$O$_2$I	412
SVR	1254	$\dot{V}$O$_2$I	84
SVRI	2061		

Seventeen hours later the situation has improved. The cardiac index and mean arterial pressure are acceptable. The systemic vascular resistance remains normal although the high wedge pressure (PCWP) has increased from 14 to 24 mmHg. An infusion of intravenous nitrates was used to correct this. The oxygen delivery and consumption remain low. The patient recovered.

Table 11 Shoemaker's hypothesis

Shoemaker's supranormal goals	Normal values
Cardiac index >50% normal >4.5/min/m^2	2.5–4 l/min/m^2
$\dot{D}$O$_2$I >600mls/min/m^2	520–720 ml/min/m^2
$\dot{V}$O$_2$I >170 mls/min/m^2	100–180 ml/min/m^2
Blood volume + 500ml	

Definitions:

Cardiac index (CI) = Cardiac output (CO) /Body surface area
Oxygen Delivery ($\dot{D}$O$_2$I) = CI × CaO$_2$ × 10 where CaO$_2$ is the arterial oxygen content.
Oxygen consumption ($\dot{V}$O$_2$I) = CI × (CaO$_2$ – C$\overline{v}$O$_2$) × 10.

This work suggests that if these supranormal goals can be achieved a dramatic reduction in mortality can be achieved.

THE 'G' SUIT

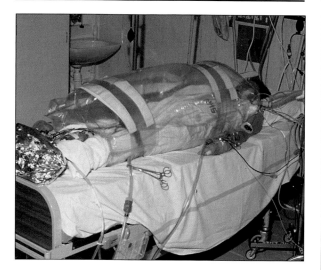

Fig. 184 The suit was specifically designed to aid the stabilisation of bleeding abdominal aneurysms. It is bulky when inflated and compromises respiration unless the patient is being mechanically ventilated, and it prohibits access. However, it is the safest way to transfer such patients to the operating theatre. Other similar devices are available.

ABDOMINAL DRAIN

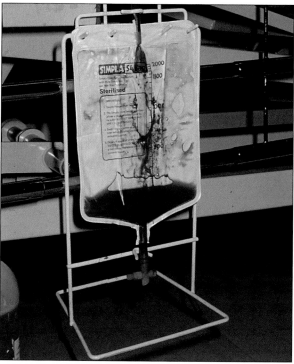

Fig. 185 Measuring abdominal losses via the drains is misleading, as drains can become blocked.

INTRA-ABDOMINAL CATASTROPHE

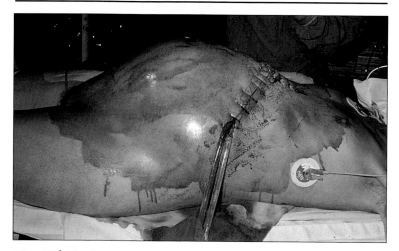

Fig. 186 The large increase in abdominal girth is a sure sign that massive haemorrhage has occurred. The surgeon must return the patient to theatre as soon as possible. Note that the drains failed to prevent blood accumulating in the abdomen.

Chapter 2 **Respiratory care in the ICU**

GENERAL

Fig. 187 Acute respiratory failure can be defined as life-threatening hypoxia or hypercapnia. Clinical examination can be misleading. An arterial blood gas is sometimes needed to confirm the diagnosis. A PaO_2 <8 kPa (60 mmHg) breathing room air or a $PaCO_2$ >6.5 kPa (50 mmHg) and a pH <7.30 (H^+<50 nmol/l) are values which cause concern. There are many causes, and the main ones are summarised in **Table 12**.

The speed of onset may preclude a detailed assessment but an increasing respiratory rate >35/min is ominous. A patient cannot cough with an FRC below 1.5 litres or sleep with an FRC less than 0.8 litres.

ACUTE RESPIRATORY FAILURE

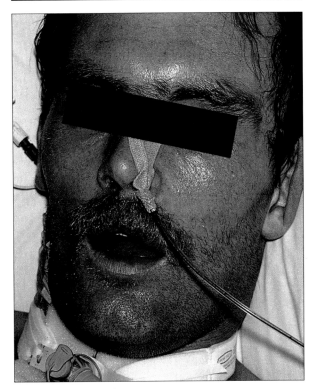

Fig. 187 Typical facies.

Table 12 Some causes of respiratory failure

Central nervous system	Respiratory obstruction	Acute/chronic lung disease	Neuromuscular
Drugs	Asthma	Chronic bronchitis	Myasthenia
Head injury	Epiglottitis	Pneumonia	Guillain–Barré
Tumour	Tumour	Inhalation	Polio
Infection	Foreign body	Aspiration	Myotonia
Cerebral accident	Gross obesity	ARDS	Tetanus
		Cystic fibrosis	Dystrophy
		Drugs	
		Occupational	
		Interstitial	
		Myopathy	

Metabolic failure	Other
Endocrine	Chest injury
Pancreatitis	Kyphoscoliosis
Hepatic	Tetraplegia
Renal	Sepsis
Low potassium	
Low phosphate	
Hyperglycaemia	

MISPLACED OROTRACHEAL TUBE

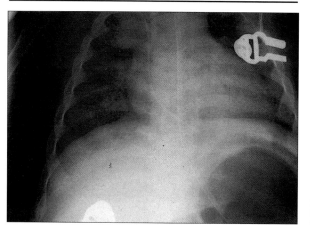

Fig. 188 This tracheal tube has been placed in the oesophagus. Realising that something was wrong the anaesthetist ventilated the lungs with a mask. The earlier attempt at ventilation lead to gross distention of the stomach.

CHEST RADIOGRAPH OF RESPIRATORY COMPROMISE

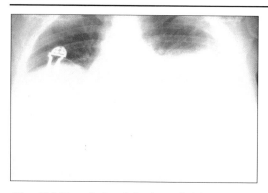

Fig. 190 Very little of the lung fields are seen on this radiograph. Diaphragmatic descent is prevented by the tense ascites.

SHOCK

Fig. 192 Early stabilisation of the cardiorespiratory systems is crucial to successfully treat the shocked patient.

GROSS ASCITES

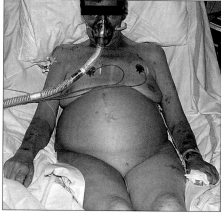

Fig. 189 This patient cannot breathe if laid flat because the ascites push the diaphragm up.

POST-THORACOTOMY

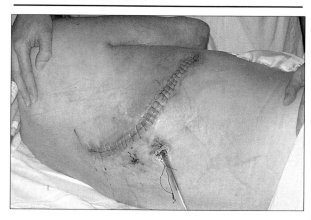

Fig. 191 A stormy period of adjustment may follow lung surgery. Lung volumes are diminished by up to 40%. Good analgesia is important to ensure adequate coughing, movement and deep breathing.

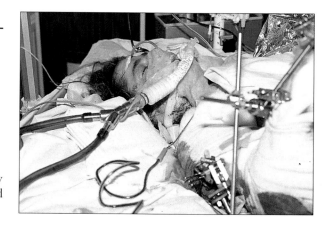

COMA: DRUG POISONING

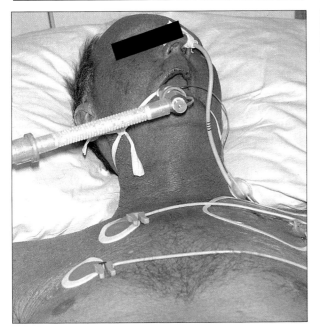

Fig. 193 A central cause of respiratory failure.

LEFT PNEUMOTHORAX

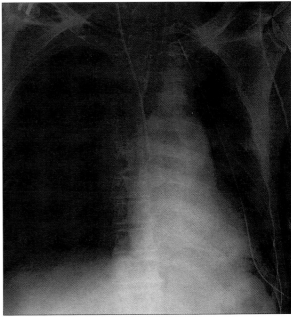

Fig. 194 A large left pneumothorax is seen on this chest radiograph. A chest drain has been inserted but the lung has not re-expanded. A compensatory increase in the size of the right lung has occurred.

LOBAR PNEUMONIA

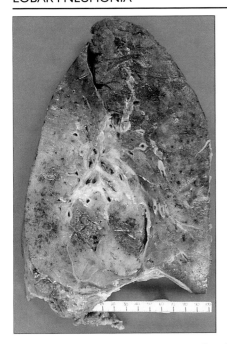

Fig. 195 A severe lobar pneumonia has led to exhaustion and collapse, needing mechanical ventilation.

CYSTIC FIBROSIS

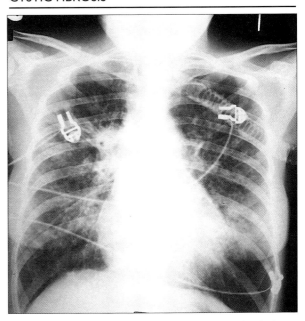

Fig. 196 A chest radiograph shows that both lung fields are fibrotic.

CLUBBING

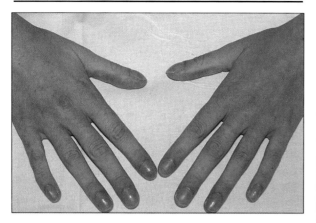

Fig. 197 The normal angle between fingernail and nail base is approximately 160°. In clubbing this angle straightens out and later becomes visibly swollen. In this case it is a feature of chronic hypoxia.

ACUTE RESPIRATORY FAILURE IN CHRONIC OBSTRUCTIVE AIRWAYS DISEASE

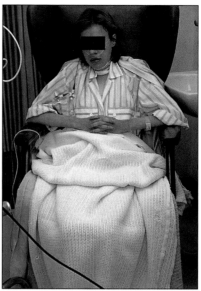

Fig. 198 In chronic conditions, prolonged hypoxia (see **Fig. 197**) leads to polycythaemia. These patients prefer to spend their night-time sitting in chairs as the FRC is better maintained. This woman was chair-bound; her exercise tolerance was limited. Measurement of blood gases showed a normal pH with a PaO_2 of 8 kPa (62 mmHg) and a $PaCO_2$ of 8 kPa (62 mmHg). To compensate for her respiratory acidosis there is a metabolic alkalosis with a bicarbonate of 40 mmol/l.

ABDOMINAL RESPIRATION

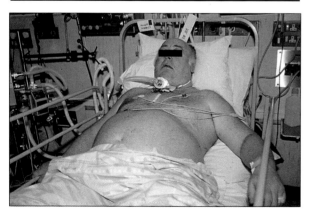

Fig. 199 This patient had predominantly diaphragmatic respiration, which impairs normal lateral respiratory excursion. A panting, 'frog-like', unco-ordinated effort is made.

ASYMMETRICAL CHEST MOVEMENT

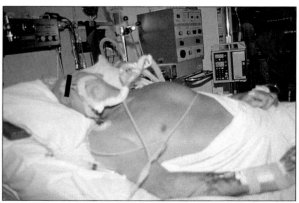

Fig. 200 The left side of the chest is overinflating. There is a misplaced tracheal tube in the left main bronchus.

AIRWAY OBSTRUCTION: HAEMANGIOMA

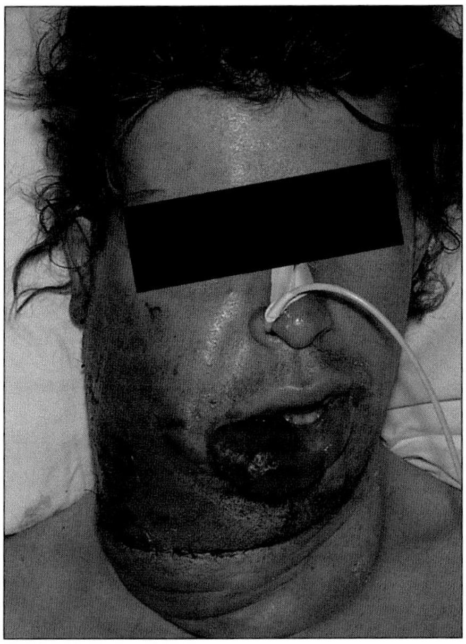

AIRWAY OBSTRUCTION: ACUTE TONSILLITIS

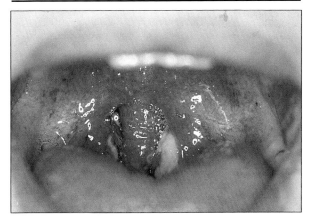

Fig. 202 Virtually total occlusion of the airway by tonsillar enlargement.

Fig. 201 This man presented with a haemangioma of the neck and face. On lying flat his airway obstructed, which was relieved by sitting forward. The haemangioma extended down into his pharynx.

STRIDOR: FUNGATING TUMOUR OF THE LARYNX

BLEEDING AFTER THYROIDECTOMY

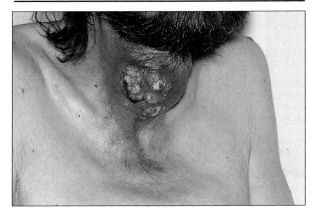

Fig. 203 The trachea is narrowed to less than 4 mm. This produces stridor.

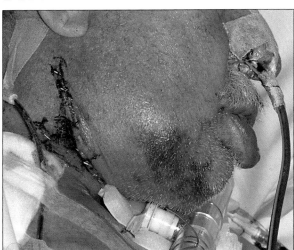

Fig. 204 This complication of thyroidectomy causes life-threatening airway obstruction. Removal of the skin clips allows the neck to distend anteriorly, but the anatomy of the larynx is usually so distorted as to challenge the anaesthetist's skill.

OXYGEN THERAPY

Most respiratory failure results primarily in hypoxia (type 1). This is amenable to oxygen therapy. Sufficient oxygen to reach an arterial oxygen saturation of at least 90% is the goal.

The presence of hypercapnia (type 2) should raise the possibility of oxygen sensitivity seen in chronic lung disease. Too much oxygen in these situations will be detrimental but the patient's life is still in jeopardy from hypoxia. Hypercapnia may also occur in type 1 respiratory failure as a pre-terminal event.

OXIMETER

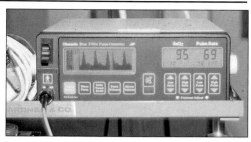

Fig. 205 Simple and quick monitoring of tissue oxygen levels (SpO_2) can now be undertaken at the bedside continuously using oximeters. This is a routine item used on every patient in the ICU.

FINGER PEG

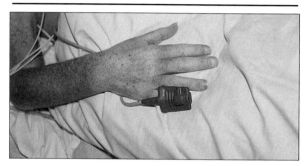

Fig. 206 A simple check on SpO_2 can be made in the majority of patients using a finger peg.

EAR-CLIP

Fig. 207 The limit-ation of oximeters is that they work poorly in cold and cyanosed limbs, but an ear-clip offers an alter-native and is useful also in children and restless adults.

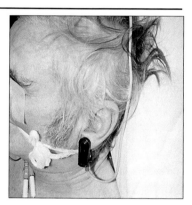

OXYGEN DISSOCIATION CURVE

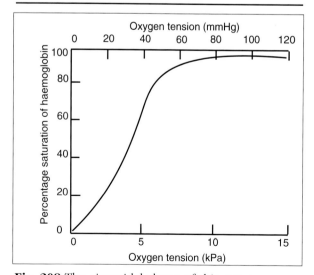

Fig. 208 The sigmoidal shape of this curve ensures that in the vertical part of the curve a small increase in oxygen tension results in a large increase in oxygen saturation in the critical clinical range.

VENOUS OXYGEN SATURATION

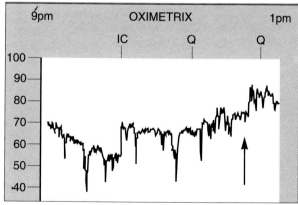

Fig. 209 This patient is profoundly desaturated; an improvement occurs when the inspired oxygen is increased to >0.8. Normal values:
Venous O_2 tension   5–5.6 kPa   37–42 mmHg
Venous O_2 content 6.7–7.2 mmol/l   15–16 vol%
Venous saturation   75%.

OXYGEN FACE MASKS

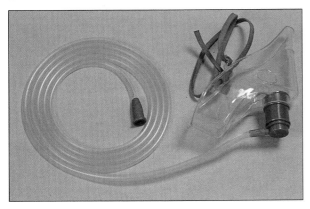
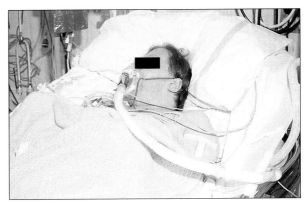

Figs 210 and **211** A close-fitting mask delivering a high F_IO_2 is suitable for routine care.

CONTROLLED OXYGEN MASK

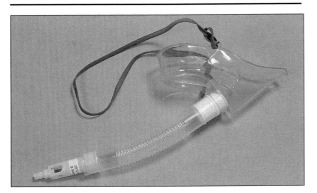

Fig. 212 When accurate control of oxygen delivery is needed, e.g. a COPD patient dependent on the hypoxic drive for ventilation, a special Venturi-based mask is required.

OXYGEN FACE TENT

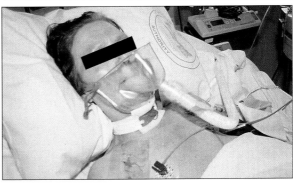

Fig. 213 An oxygen tent is comfortable to wear when inspired O_2 levels are not too important.

NASAL OXYGEN CANNULA

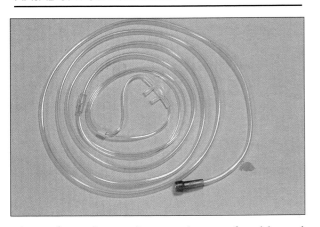

Fig. 214 Nasal cannulae are also comfortable and permit eating. They should not be used with an oxygen flow over 2 l/min or when a low F_IO_2 is needed.

FACIAL CPAP

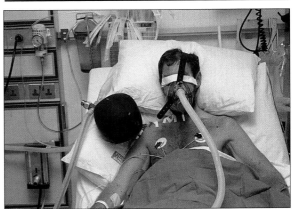

Fig. 215 Another method of supporting oxygenation is facial CPAP. It is cumbersome and time-consuming to get the mask position right, but worth persevering with. It can sometimes avoid the need for ventilation.

PHYSIOTHERAPY AND POSTURE

PHYSIOTHERAPY: VIBRATION AND PERCUSSION

Fig. 216 The physiotherapist has a key role in chest management. Vibration and percussion to the chest should be performed routinely at least twice a day on every ICU patient. In specific conditions postural drainage will precede treatment. 'Bagging' is also used to provide deep breaths and cough simulation.

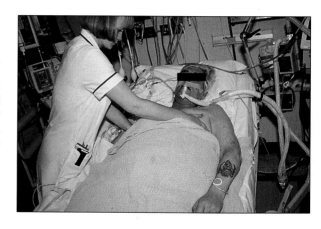

CLOSED SUCTION SYSTEM

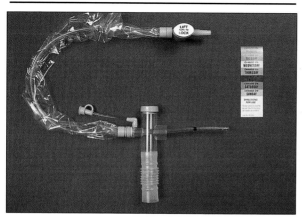

Fig. 217 The patient does not have to be disconnected from the ventilator for suction to be performed. This is a safe method for the nurses. It can be used in the intubated, spontaneously breathing patient.

BIRD VENTILATOR

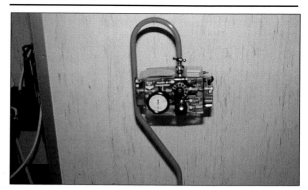

Fig. 218 This is a useful method of providing breathing exercises, using a pressurised system, in the ward and the extubated patient.

DR NELSON'S INHALER

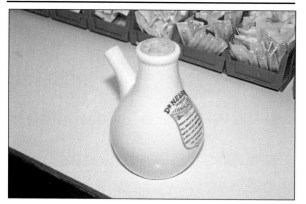

Fig. 219 Menthol crystals are dissolved in warm water in a container.

USE OF DR NELSON'S INHALER

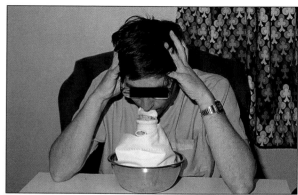

Fig. 220 The fumes are inhaled and are soothing to the airway. This is an old-fashioned but effective form of teatment.

POSTURE

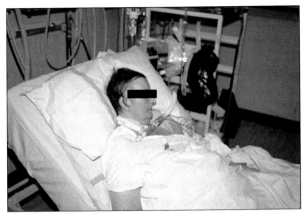

Fig. 221 Physiologically, the lungs reach maximum expansion when sitting erect.

THE PRONE POSITION

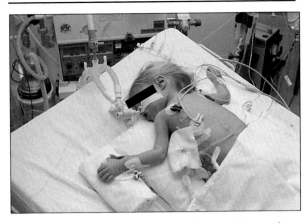

Fig. 222 It is worth considering other positions when the chest deteriorates. Despite the obvious difficulties, the prone position sometimes improves lung expansion.

ROTATIONAL THERAPY

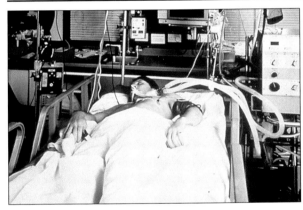

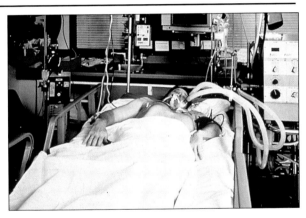

Fig. 223 and **224** Rotational beds can continuously rock the patient from side to side and are an effective method of treating and preventing atelectasis and pneumonia. They can be particularly helpful in chest trauma.

ROTATIONAL TREATMENT: EFFECT OF $S\bar{v}O_2$

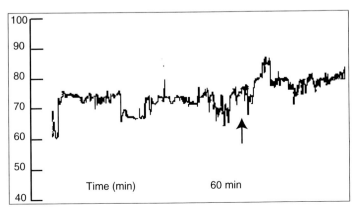

Fig. 225 A venous oximetric trace showing the onset of rotation (arrow), and the improvement within a few minutes.

TRACHEAL INTUBATION

OROTRACHEAL

Fig. 226 Useful in the short term, oral intubation tends to cause salivation and irritation. If long (un-cut) tracheal tubes are used, they may enter the right main bronchus.

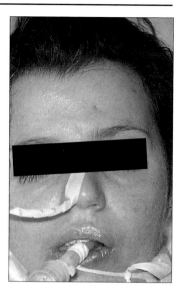

NASOTRACHEAL

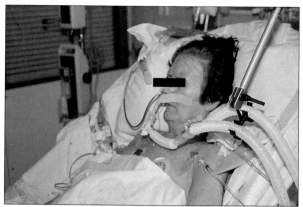

Fig. 227 This is preferred for longer-term use. An uncut tube is used to protect the external skin at the nares. Cocaine can be used to vasoconstrict the mucosa and to restrict bleeding.

Table 13 Indications for tracheal intubation

Airway obstruction
To protect the airway
Severe hypoxia
Coma
Secretion retention
To facilitate IPPV

MINITRACHEOSTOMY TUBE

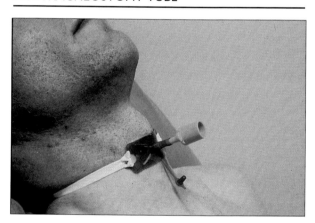

Fig. 228 The minitracheostomy tube is a 6 mm uncuffed tube placed through the cricothyroid membrane to allow suction without loss of voice. It is a simple method of dealing with secretion retention. The two major complications are incorrect placement and bleeding, but it does represent a safer option than tracheostomy.

TRACHEOSTOMY TUBE

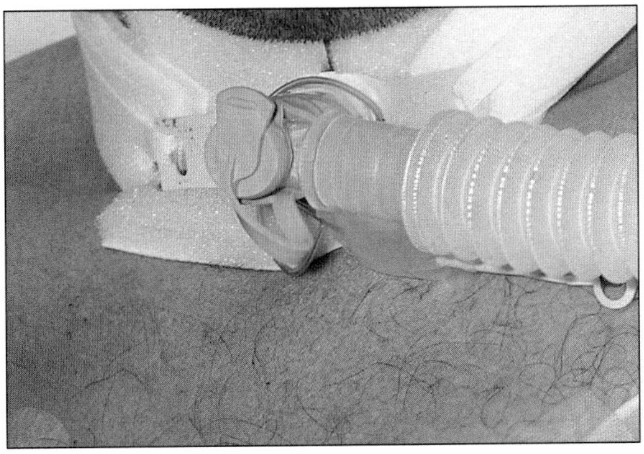

Leave the cuff inflated all the time

A foam dressing protects the skin

Humidify

Advise on 'lost voice'

Suction regularly

Fig. 229 Longer-term airway management is undertaken with a tracheostomy. It offers some advantages in terms of comfort, ease of tracheal toilet and a reduction in dead space. Incorrect insertion, haemorrhage, emphys- ema and pneumothorax are immediate risks. Serious complications can also occur. Recent evidence suggests that percutaneous insertion is safer than surgical.

Table 14 Complications of tracheostomy

Early	Late
Misplacement	Infection
Emphysema	Stenosis
Pneumothorax	Fistula
Haemorrhage	Late haemorrhage

CELLULITIS AROUND A TRACHEOSTOMY TUBE

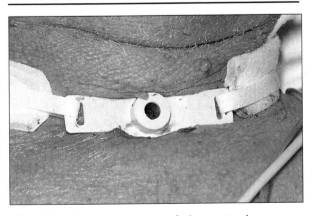

Fig. 230 Infection is one of the main long-term problems. Late haemorrhage due to vessel erosion, stenosis and fistula formation are other delayed major sequelae.

FENESTRATED TRACHEOSTOMY TUBE

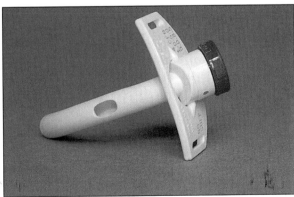

Fig. 231 It is possible to speak with a fenestrated tube *in situ*; cuffed and uncuffed versions are available. The patient must have a cough reflex.

COMMUNICATION 1

Fig. 232 Patients are frightened about losing their voices when intubated. A mobile communicator is one possible alternative means of communication.

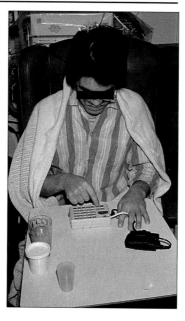

COMMUNICATION 2

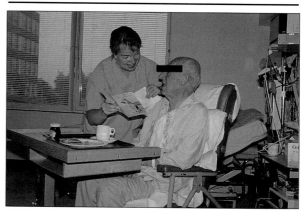

Fig. 233 Sign language, writing down words or pointing to letters are all possible forms of communication for the intubated patient.

THE NURSING TEAM 1

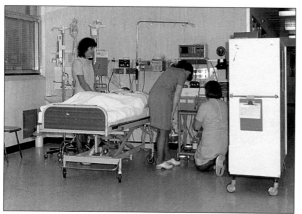

Fig. 234 The best efforts of any doctor are worthless without a highly-skilled nursing staff.

THE NURSING TEAM 2

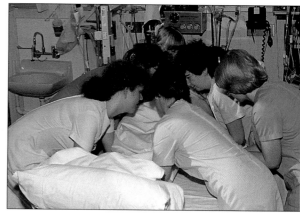

Fig. 235 The number of nurses required to care for one ICU patient has been estimated at 7.2 in every 24-hour period. If for no other reason, the cost of caring for patients in an ICU is very high.

MECHANICAL VENTILATION

Three basic approaches exist. Recreation of a negative pressure around the lungs by external means is reserved for patients with some respiratory dysfunction but with some reserve. Tracheal intubation is not needed.

Positive pressure ventilation traditionally uses a large tidal volume (Tv), with a low respiratory rate (RR), e.g. Tv 850 ml × RR 10/min.

More recently, 'jet' ventilation has been used to provide low tidal volumes and fast respiratory rates, e.g. Tv 100 ml × RR 100/min.

Both methods of positive pressure ventilation have their advocates: the traditional method relies on the large tidal volume preventing lung collapse but at the expense of producing a high intrathoracic pressure.

The 'jet' avoids this but at the expense of the functional residual capacity (FRC), so it requires positive end expiratory pressure (PEEP, see **Fig. 330**, p. 94) to help overcome this.

IRON LUNG

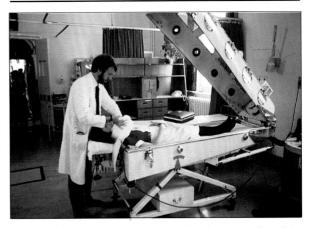

Fig. 236 The body from the neck down is placed in the tank. Polio resulting in respiratory failure is often treated this way.

CUIRASS VENTILATION

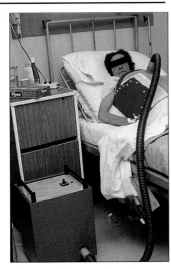

Fig. 237 The use of body shells that can be strapped on, like a waistcoat, permits some independence and mobility, and provides useful overnight ventilatory assistance. Slowly deteriorating neuromuscular disorders do well with this type of ventilation.

POSITIVE PRESSURE VENTILATION (IPPV)

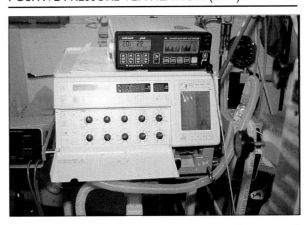

Fig. 238 Modern ventilators provide a wide range of possibilities including volume and pressure-cycled approaches. They have sophisticated oxygen, pressure, volume and disconnection alarms.

Patients commonly 'fight' the ventilator for four reasons — hypoxia, hypercapnia, acidosis and pain. If these can be reversed then it is unusual to need muscle relaxants to maintain adequate ventilation.

BACK-UP VENTILATOR: WATERS' BAG

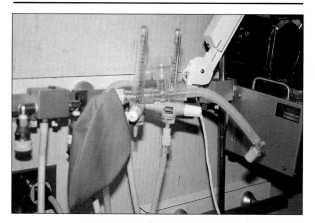

Fig. 239 Beside every bed area there must be a manual system to take over in case of ventilator failure. Vigilance is needed as ventilator failure is unpredictable.

JET VENTILATION

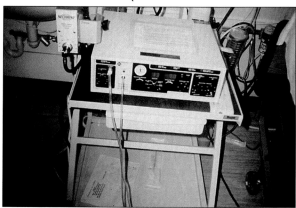

Fig. 240 Jet ventilation is especially useful in cases of bronchopleural fistula, ARDS and intractable weaning.

JET BAFFLE

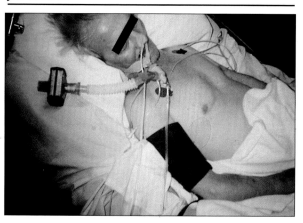

Fig. 241 This simple baffle using an airway filter reduces the noise of the jet ventilator considerably.

WEANING

POSTOPERATIVE CASES

Successful weaning requires a haemodynamically stable patient with a low oxygen requirement (F_IO_2 <0.5) who is afebrile and nourished. There is no single way to wean every patient. It can be quick, taking perhaps an hour the day after major surgery, or many days if the patient has a long, debilitating illness.

Straightforward patients can often go on to a T-piece system after showing their ability to breathe. If the step down to a T piece is too soon, a CPAP circuit is often the answer.

WRIGHT'S RESPIROMETER

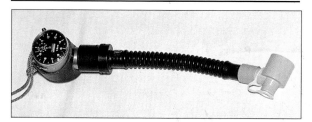

Fig. 242 A reasonable tidal volume of >350 ml/breath with a rate below 30 breaths/min and the ability to sustain this are usually needed.

GILSTON'S T PIECE

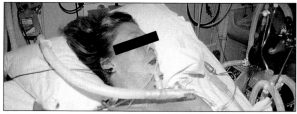

Fig. 243 The simplest method of withdrawing the ventilator is to transfer onto the lightweight T piece. Blood gases, a qualitative method of assessment, should be performed after 20 min and then as indicated every 1–2 hours.

DEBILITATED PATIENTS: WEANING USING THE VENTILATOR

There are two approaches in less predictable situations. First, the stronger patient can be allowed to breathe using the machine to help (pressure support or assist mode) for periods of 1–2 hours and then rested and the cycle repeated for increasing periods. It is important that the patient is not pushed to the point of exhaustion. These patients often need PEEP added to the circuit to sustain the FRC.

CPAP CONTROLS

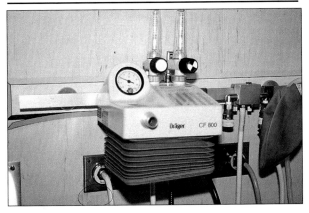

Fig. 245 The flow rate and inspired oxygen content can be varied.

CHARTING

To manage and organise the care of ICU patients safely, careful record keeping must be undertaken.

CHARTS

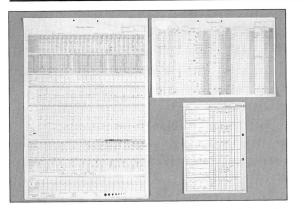

Fig. 247 These are examples of three of the charts used in every admission, namely fluid balance with results attached; a haemodynamic/respiratory care chart and a prescription chart.

CPAP BELLOWS

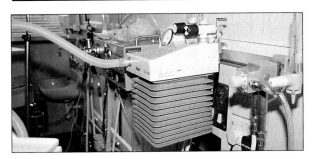

Fig. 244 To recruit and maintain FRC when weaning from the ventilator or as a separate ventilatory support, the CPAP bellows can be useful. An air/oxygen flow is drawn from the bellows.

CPAP VALVE

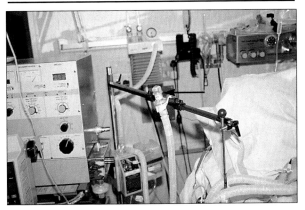

Fig. 246 The CPAP valve is placed vertically (arrow) and set between 3 and 10 cmH$_2$O. As the patient gets stronger the level can be reduced.

COMPUTER RECORDS

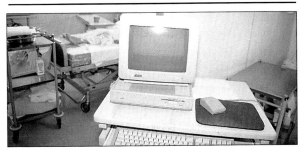

Fig. 248 An alternative is to record all information onto a computer which will generate its own record. The computer can also be used to control various infusions of drugs and fluid.

DAILY WORK PLAN

FREEMAN HOSPITAL N.H.S. TRUST

GENERAL INTENSIVE THERAPY UNIT

DAILY WORK PLAN   SHEET NO:_____   DATE:_____   WARD ROUND WITH DR._____

PATIENT DETAILS:	**DIAGNOSIS:**

CURRENT PROBLEMS	**CHANGES IN LAST 24 HOURS**

CARDIOVASCULAR	**RESPIRATORY** DRUGS
CPK	
DRUGS	
ECHO	**SR/ CMV/ SIMV/ ASSIST/ CPAP/ HFJV**
ECG	BLOOD GASES

NEUROLOGICAL **GCS Score:**	**ABDOMINAL** NG Losses Drains
Sleep	
Sedation	
Other Drugs	Amylase PT Antacid:
Skin Care	Nutrition - NG/IV

MICROBIOLOGY Temp °C	**FLUID BALANCE**
Micro-organism Antibiotic Date Site 1 2 3 4 5	Renal Function
Lines in Situ Site When Inserted Arterial - Central - Peripheral -	Drugs

INVESTIGATIONS ORDERED	**DAILY PLAN**
FBC **LFT** **CULTURES** **U & E** **Ca++** **-Blood** **Clotting** **Mg++** **-Sputum** **CXR** **Phosphate** **-Urine** **USS** **CT Scan**	

SIGNATURE OF RESIDENT:

AKS/CB/GITU

Fig. 249 Straightforward management can be handled with a work plan that permits a rapid review of care and sets out the day's aims. As with all notes, it should be signed and dated. The time of other entries should be recorded.

CHEST DISORDERS

Four conditions dominate ICU chest care in the critically ill: pneumonia; aspiration; atelectasis and pulmonary oedema (see **Fig. 350**, p. 102). Acute exacerbations of chronic lung disease are regular features with, less frequently, interstitial lung disease.

PNEUMONIA

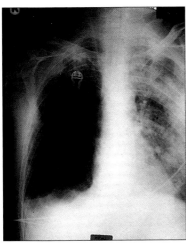

Fig. 250 In this patient an exacerbation of COPD was brought on by *Streptococcus pneumonia*.

In other patients, tracheal intubation makes them vulnerable to the development of pneumonia, as the normal protective mechanisms of the respiratory tract have been bypassed.

Another factor contributing to pneumonia is the neutralising of gastric pH with H_2 antagonists to prevent stress ulcers. This leads to bacterial colonisation of the stomach, with an increase in nosocomial pneumonia.

Community-acquired infections also occur. They are commonly caused by *Streptococcus pneumonia*, *Haemophilus influenza* and anaerobes. In hospital-acquired infections, Gram-negative organisms dominate. Annual immunisation against influenza is helpful.

Fig. 252 This patient was unwell the morning after abdominal surgery, and was clearly in respiratory failure and exhausted. He has collapsed the left lung. He was stabilised on a ventilator and adequate oxygenation achieved before bronchoscopy was undertaken. Patients like this do not do well unless this approach is used.

Anticipation of this problem can save life. Early physiotherapy coupled with a minitracheostomy (see **Fig. 228**, p. 64) in appropriate situations can prevent further deterioration.

This is a well-recognised complication after surgery and in patients who produce a lot of secretions, such as those with cystic fibrosis or a chest infection.

ASPIRATION: MENDELSON'S SYNDROME

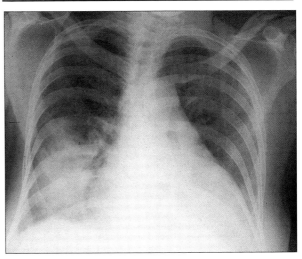

Fig. 251 This patient has inhaled gastric contents (Mendelson's syndrome), resulting in a life-threatening collapse. Hypoxia, bronchospasm, cyanosis and respiratory insufficiency will rapidly cause death.

Other substances sometimes aspirate include water (near drowning), blood, foreign bodies, nasogastric feed and contrast material.

ATELECTASIS

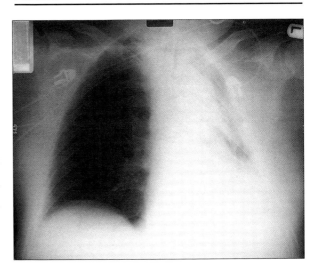

TUBERCULOSIS

Fig. 253 Tuberculosis is a condition associated with malnutrition, alcoholism, and immunosuppression. It is more often seen in Asian, Eskimo, Indian and black communities. Although it is an 'old' disease, it should always be thought about in patients at risk.

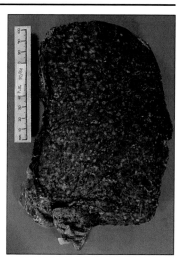

ASTHMA: PEAK-FLOW METER

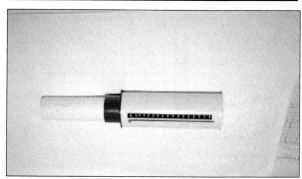

Fig. 254 The peak-flow meter permits an easy bedside test. A level below 80 l/min is perilous.

ASTHMA: SPIROMETRY

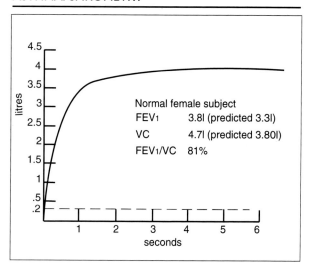

Normal female subject
FEV$_1$ 3.8l (predicted 3.3l)
VC 4.7l (predicted 3.80l)
FEV$_1$/VC 81%

Fig. 255 If the patient is less incapacitated, spirometry will reveal the degree of airway obstruction, and whether it is reversible.

SEVERE AIRWAYS OBSTRUCTION

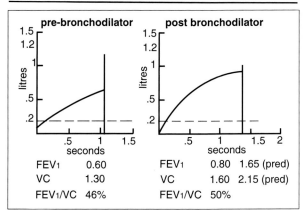

pre-bronchodilator
FEV$_1$ 0.60
VC 1.30
FEV$_1$/VC 46%

post bronchodilator
FEV$_1$ 0.80 1.65 (pred)
VC 1.60 2.15 (pred)
FEV$_1$/VC 50%

Fig. 256 There is a small reversible element here.

STATUS ASTHMATICUS

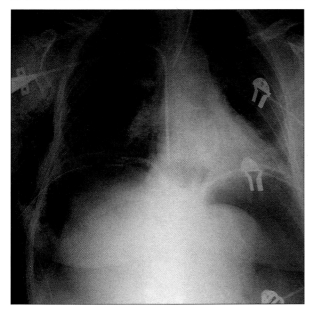

Fig. 257 Surgical emphysema and free abdominal gas in an asthmatic on a ventilator with unremitting bronchospasm. This is a very dangerous situation.

A small percentage (<3%) of asthmatics will require ventilation. There often has been a period of un-recognised deterioration and increasingly futile medication. Exhaustion, hypoxia, unrelieved broncho-spasm and cardiovascular collapse will inevitably result in a respiratory arrest, unless intervention occurs.

NEBULISER

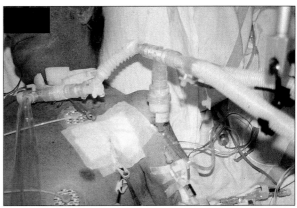

Fig. 258 Bronchodilators can be delivered through a tracheal tube. Many intubated patients develop bronchospasm because of the tracheal tube.

NEBULISER COMPONENTS

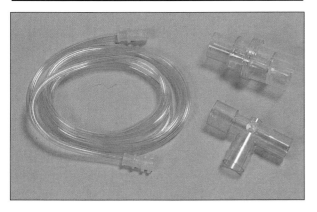

Fig. 259 Certain drugs, notably antibiotics, block the nebuliser so always check this possibility first.

COR PULMONALE: BLUE BLOATER

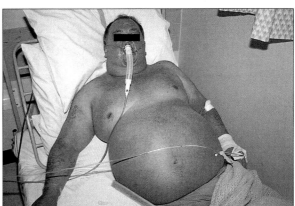

Fig. 260 The presentation of a patient with hypoxaemia, carbon dioxide retention and right heart failure (cor pulmonale) is a feature of severe restrictive respiratory disease.

SPIROMETRY IN RESTRICTIVE DISEASE

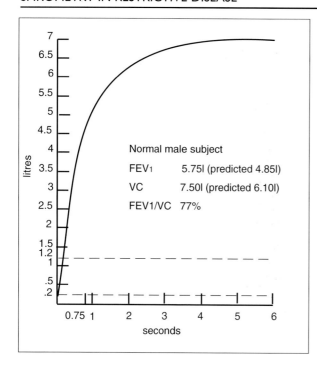

Normal male subject

FEV₁   5.75l (predicted 4.85l)

VC   7.50l (predicted 6.10l)

FEV1/VC 77%

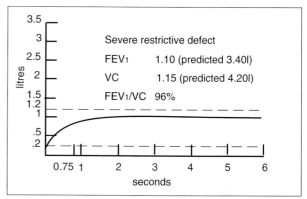

Severe restrictive defect

FEV₁   1.10 (predicted 3.40l)

VC   1.15 (predicted 4.20l)

FEV1/VC 96%

Figs 261 and **262** The spirometry shows small lungs with a low volume and capacity.

BULLA

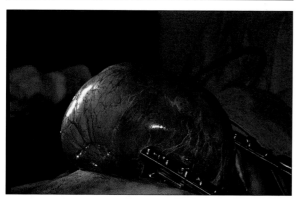

Figs 263 and **264** Huge bullae are associated with emphysema.

CT SCAN OF BULLA

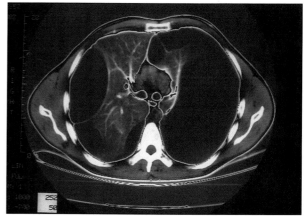

EMPHYSEMA: PINK PUFFER

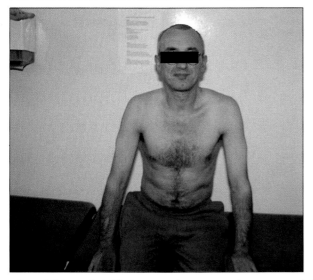 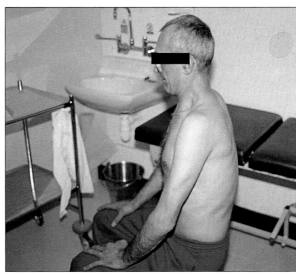

Figs 265 and **266** Severe dyspnoea, but normal blood gases characterise emphysema. This patient could not walk ten metres.

BRONCHOPLEURAL FISTULA

PLEURAL EFFUSION

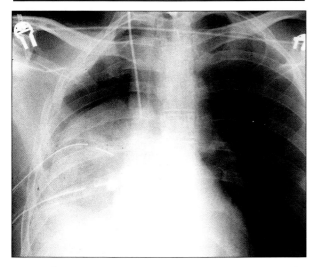 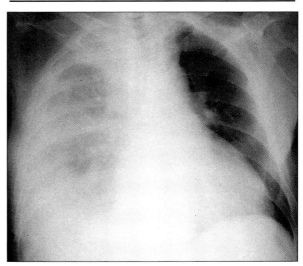

Fig. 267 This lung has failed to expand despite the presence of two chest drains. It was associated with an empyema.

Fig. 268 Accumulation of fluid in the right pleural space. Its location is best identified with an ultrasound scan.

TAPPING THE CHEST

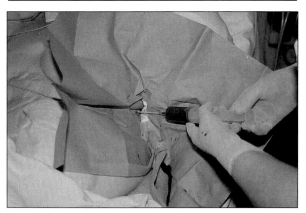

Fig. 269 The effusion (see **Fig. 268**, p. 75) can be drained by a single drainage procedure.

BLOOD-STAINED EFFUSION

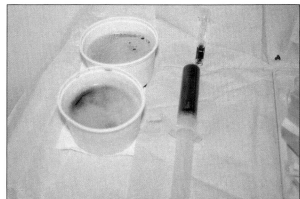

Fig. 270 This blood-stained effusion is secondary to pneumonia. A sample should be sent for culture and malignant cells.

EMPYEMA

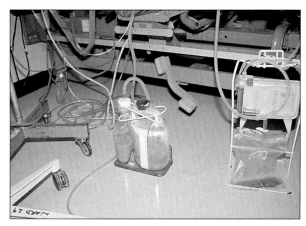

Fig. 271 Purulent fluid draining from the pleural cavity.

CHEST RADIOGRAPH OF EMPYEMA

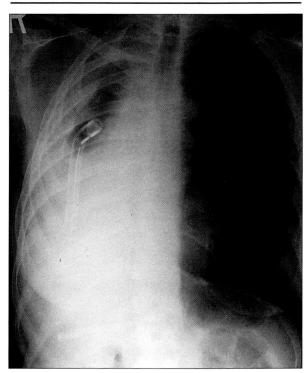

Fig. 272 A chest full of pus with very little lung expanded. The drain acts like an overflow cistern in this case.

REPEATED CHEST DRAINS

Fig. 273 This patient had to have numerous chest drains inserted to drain her empyema.

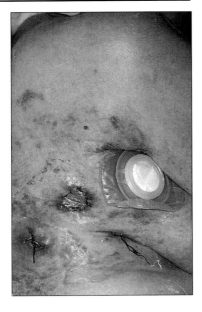

THE LUNG IN ADULT RESPIRATORY DISTRESS SYNDROME (ARDS)

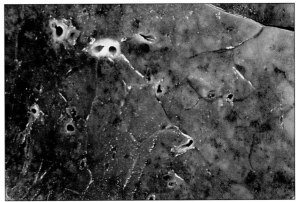

Fig. 274 Typically triggered by sepsis, trauma or aspiration of gastric contents. The initial phase is acute inflammation, with neutrophilia and fluid leakage. If the lung does not recover, a relentless fibrotic process occurs (see **Fig 275** below and **Fig. 308**, p. 86).

HISTOLOGY IN ARDS

Fig. 275 This biopsy was taken seven days after paraquat ingestion. The hyaline membranes are seen resolving. The cuboidal-type cells characteristic of the repair process are present.

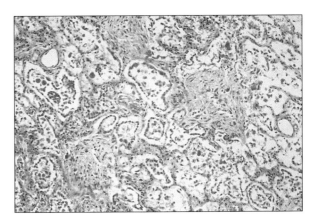

SCOLIOSIS

Fig. 276 This characteristic spinal deformity will result in respiratory failure. Patients with scoliosis may need intensive care after operations because of their difficulty in breathing.

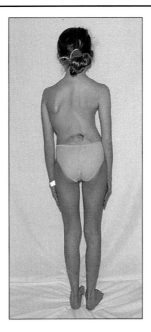

Fig. 277 Scoliosis, which causes restriction on one side and compensatory over-distension of the other side of the chest wall, often occurs in association with kyphosis (see **Fig. 278** below and **Fig. 291**, p. 82).

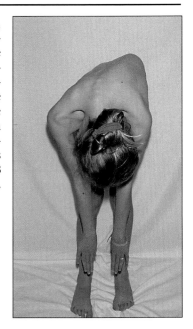

KYPHOSIS

Fig. 278 Kyphosis is another potential cause of respiratory failure.

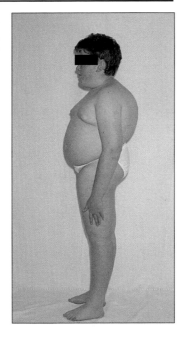

Chapter 3 **The role of radiology**

INTRODUCTION

Radiology can help with diagnosis in the seriously ill patient. At the bedside portable films, ultrasound and echocardiography can be performed. Despite the need to transport the critically ill patient to the X-Ray Department for some procedures such as screening of central lines, pacemaker insertion, angiography, venography and CT scanning, this is usually a safe and practical proposition. It does require planning, portable ventilation and monitoring equipment and a screening room designed with these needs in mind.

PNEUMOPERICARDIUM

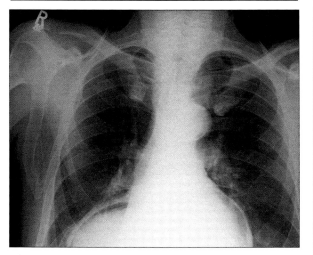

Fig. 279 Pneumopericardium.

BILATERAL PNEUMOTHORAX

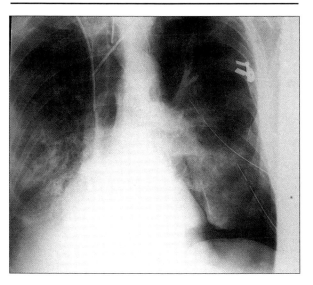

Fig. 281 Bilateral pneumothorax.

PNEUMOTHORAX

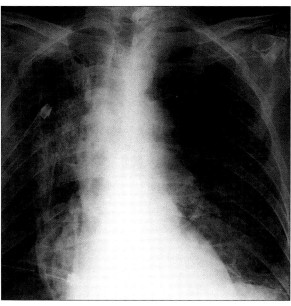

Fig. 280 Pneumothorax after fracture of two ribs. Of concern is the failure to re-expand the lung despite the presence of three chest drains.

RIGHT PNEUMOTHORAX

Fig. 282 This was caused by the insertion of an internal jugular line and is a well-recognised complication of central line insertion. The sub-clavian route is more of a risk (1%) than the internal jugular route (0.05%) but in practice the experience and skill of the operator is often the determining factor.

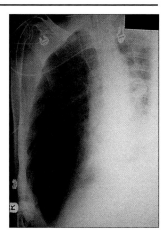

GROSS SURGICAL EMPHYSEMA

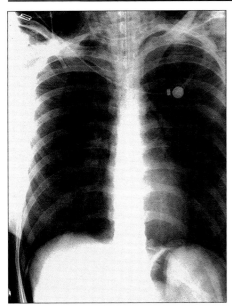

Fig. 283 This patient had acute asthma with generalised surgical emphysema. Air has tracked down from the chest to produce air under the diaphragm. This may mislead the clinician to believe there is perforated viscera.

GROSS GASTRIC DISTENSION AFTER CARDIAC ARREST

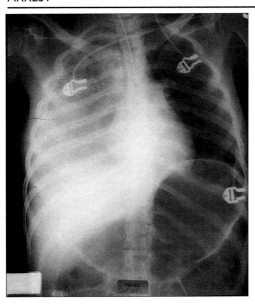

Fig. 285 Immediately after a cardiac arrest this patient was ventilated using a 'bag and mask'. This inflated not only the lungs, but also the stomach. After successful tracheal intubation the patient remained difficult to ventilate because of the gastric distention. Severe hypoxia occurred. The patient has also aspirated stomach contents into the right lung during the resuscitation, which is common.

ACUTE PERFORATION OF AN ABDOMINAL VISCUS

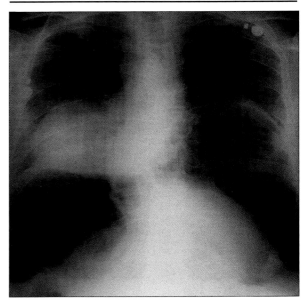

Fig. 284 Free air in the abdominal cavity is usually seen in an erect chest X-ray under the diaphragm. It is usually seen after abdominal operations. However, spontaneous perforation of a viscus may occur in any critically ill patient.

MISPLACED PULMONARY ARTERY CATHETER (PAC)

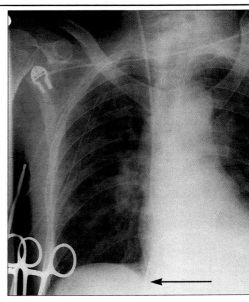

Fig. 286 The PAC has been passed into the liver (arrow). In the absence of screening facilities the clinician depends on pressure wave changes to show the progress of the catheter through the heart (see **Fig. 383**, p. 113). It would be clear that this catheter was wrongly placed, but not where it had gone until a chest radiograph was taken. Difficult placements can often be solved by using screening facilities.

INTUBATION RIGHT MAIN BRONCHUS: A 30 CM CENTRAL LINE

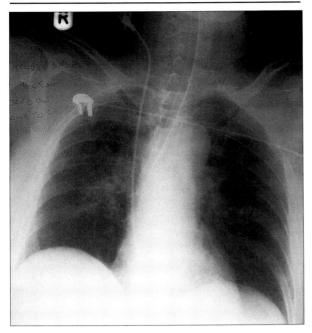

Fig. 287 The tracheal tube has been placed in the right main bronchus and is too long. This is a common finding in the ICU.

The use of a 30 cm line in the neck veins similarly has led to the line being too far into the heart. Routine chest radiographs are mandatory after such procedures to check correct placement.

LOOP IN THE PAC

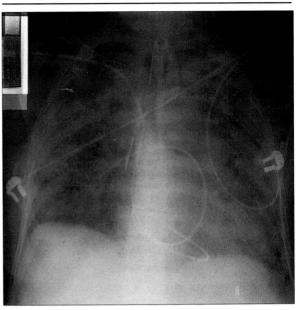

Fig. 288 Coiling, loops and occasional knots occur in the placement of PACs. They are encouraged by the length the catheter has to travel (in this case the right subclavian vein), the presence of a large right ventricle and a sluggishly beating heart.

UNUSUAL FOREIGN BODY

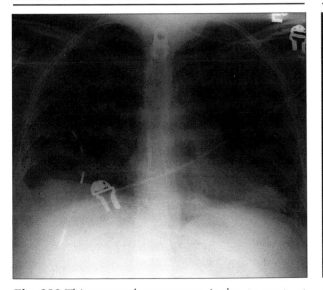

Fig. 289 This unusual appearance is due to contrast media trapped in a tube (seen as menisci) lying outside the chest.

THORACOPLASTY

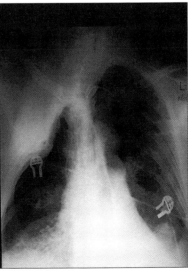

Fig. 290 Gross chest wall deformity following surgical treatment of tuberculosis.

KYPHOSCOLIOSIS

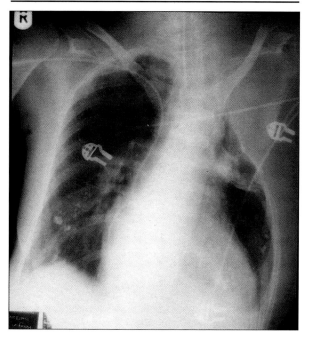

Fig. 291 Note the characteristic compensatory emphysema of the right lung with restrictive expansion of the left lung.

EMPHYSEMA

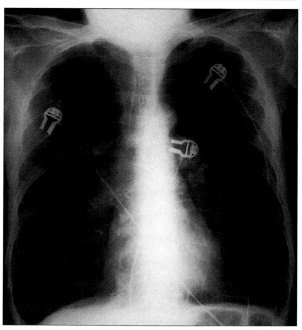

Fig. 292 Grossly distended lung fields.

HIATUS HERNIA

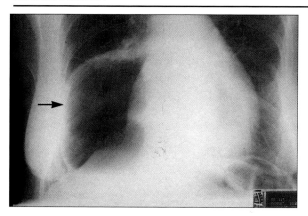

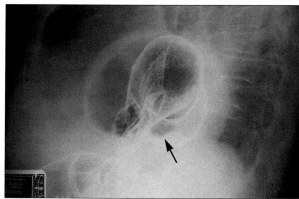

Figs 293 and **294** The anterior/posterior (**293**, left) and lateral (**294**, right) views of the chest show a significant hiatus hernia (arrows).

The AP view alone would have been misleading, perhaps suggesting a bulla. Lateral films are difficult to obtain in ICU patients, making chest film interpretation more difficult.

COLLAPSE LEFT LOWER LOBE

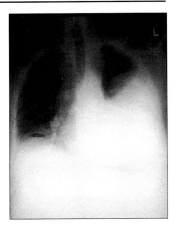

Fig. 295 This patient has developed a large effusion at the base of the left lung. An ultrasound of the chest (to demonstrate fluid and determine needle aspiration site) and of the abdomen to exclude a subphrenic collection is indicated. There is also the small air bubble under the right diaphragm, a legacy of previous abdominal surgery.

RIGHT SUBPHRENIC COLLECTION

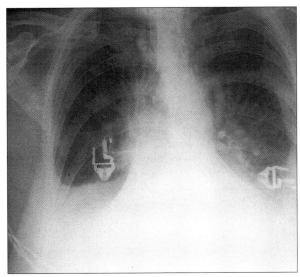

Fig. 296 This 63-year-old lady presented with a pancreatic abscess. This fluid, seen at the right base of the lung, led to an ultrasound of the abdomen being performed and a subphrenic collection being drained. *Streptococcus faecalis* was grown from the fluid aspirated.

CT SCAN OF SUBPHRENIC ABSCESS

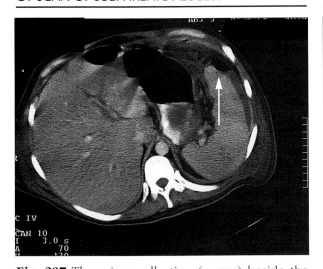

Fig. 297 There is a collection (arrow) beside the spleen with a gas bubble present. This was sampled and *Escherichia coli* grown. It resolved with antibiotics. Subphrenic collections are less common than previously, largely because of a better understanding of antibiotic therapy.

MULTIPLE ABDOMINAL ABSCESSES

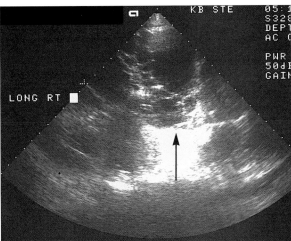

Fig. 298 This ultrasound of the abdomen shows multiloculated collections (arrow), surrounding fixed small bowel and clear peritoneal fluid.

RIGHT LUNG ASPIRATION

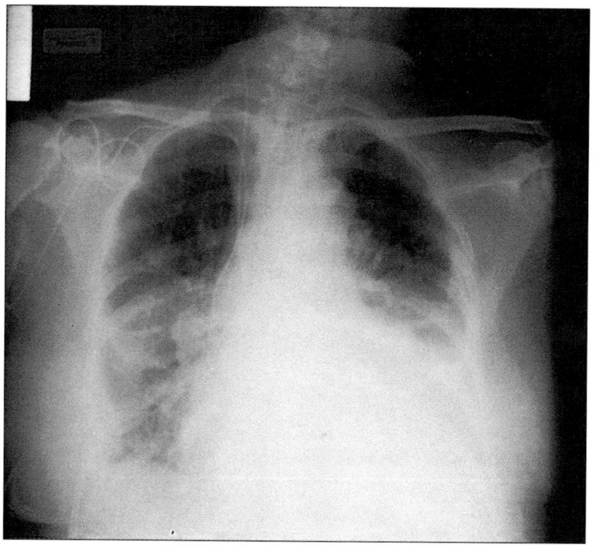

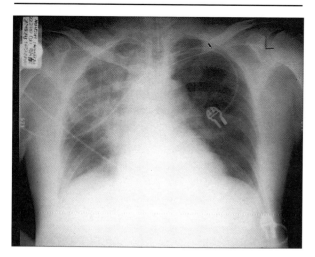

Fig. 299 The classic site of aspiration is into the right lung, the right main bronchus is only 2 in long and with a narrow angle off the trachea (25°). As little as 30 ml of gastric acid with a pH <2.5 can result in life-threatening chemical pneumonia.

LEFT LUNG ASPIRATION

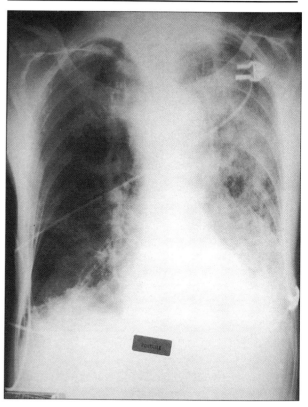

Fig. 300 Left-sided aspiration of gastric contents can occur, but is less common.

RIGHT LOBAR PNEUMONIA

Fig. 301 Early sputum collection and blood cultures are helpful in determining the causative organism. Protected bronchial washings may also be required.

LEFT BRONCHOPNEUMONIA

RIGHT UPPER AND MIDDLE LOBE PNEUMONIA

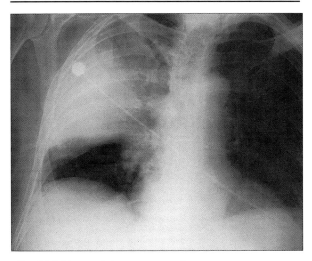

Fig. 302 This 43-year-old man underwent cystectomy for bladder cancer. He later developed a large bowel fistula, an *Escherichia coli* septicaemia and broncho-pneumonia. This took 27 days to resolve. Note also the left internal jugular line is incorrectly placed in the azygos vein.

Fig. 303 Upper lobe pneumonias are more common in tuberculosis and *Klebsiella* infections.

BILATERAL PLEURAL EFFUSIONS

LARGE RIGHT PLEURAL EFFUSION AFTER BILATERAL ASPIRATION

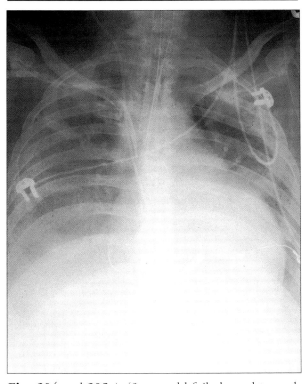

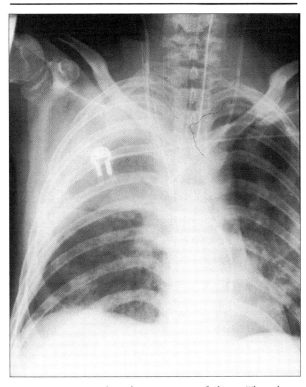

Figs 304 and **305** A 43-year-old failed renal transplant patient presented with respiratory failure. The chest radiograph showed bilateral pleural effusions. Chest aspiration, based on clinical signs, was unsuccessful. After drainage the right upper lobe collapsed. Ultrasound-guided aspiration of the chest revealed effusions of 1400 ml on the left and 700 ml on the right (the latter was probably not fully drained). When draining effusions it is better to be guided by ultrasound. The needle should be placed high rather than low.

MISPLACED CENTRAL LINE CAUSING EFFUSION

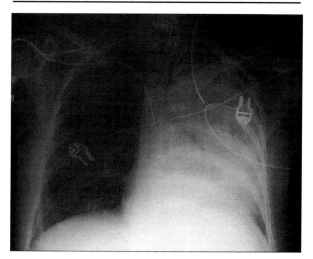

Fig. 306 This internal jugular catheter is clearly outside the normal line of insertion. Misplaced intravenous fluid has produced this effusion.

PULMONARY OEDEMA

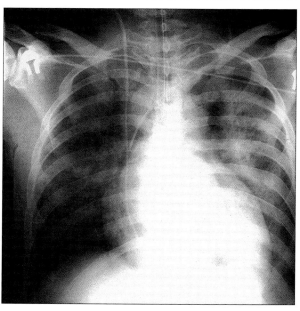

Fig. 307 Frothy blood-stained secretions pour up the airway (see **Fig. 346**, p. 100).

ARDS DUE TO SEPSIS

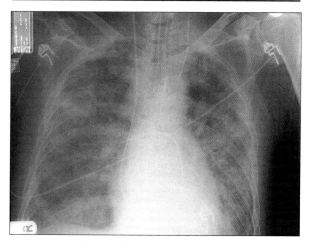

Fig. 308 Diffuse infiltrates on chest X-ray, hypoxia and a normal pulmonary wedge pressure are the features of this condition, which is called ARDS (see **Figs 274** and **275**, p. 77).

OVERTRANSFUSION CAUSING PULMONARY OEDEMA

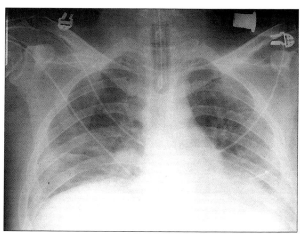

Fig. 309 This 19-year-old man received 20 units of blood after blunt trauma to the liver. He subsequently developed this chest radiograph appearance. Ventilation with an F_1O_2 and PEEP of 10 cmH$_2$O resulted in a PaO$_2$ of 10.8 kPa and a PaCO$_2$ of 5.4 kPa. The wedge pressure was 30 mmHg (normal 6–12 mmHg), confirming this was fluid overload and not ARDS.

MASSIVE COLLAPSE (WHITE OUT) LEFT LUNG

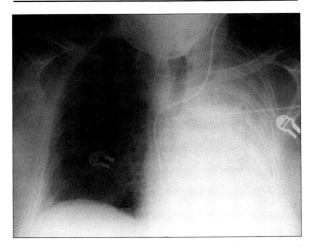

Fig. 310 This chest X-ray shows the trachea deviated to the left. A plug of mucus has occluded the left main bronchus. Fibreoptic bronchoscopy removed 50 ml of pus from this side. The patient was a 49-year-old woman with pancreatitis. She suffered a small bowel perforation and four days postoperatively was noted to have complete collapse of the left lung.

RIGID BRONCHOSCOPE

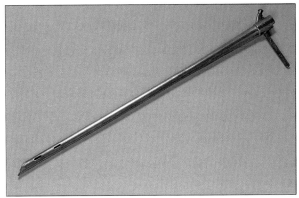

Fig. 311 The alternative to a fibreoptic bronchoscope is the rigid bronchoscope that permits large-bore suction to remove plugs. It requires the removal of the tracheal tube. Ventilatory support with additional oxygen is usually given using a Venturi system.

MASSIVE COLLAPSE OF RIGHT LUNG

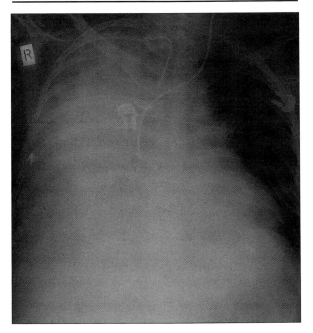

Fig. 312 Also present are multiple coils of the nasogastric tube in the stomach.

TRACHEAL TUBE CAUSING COLLAPSE

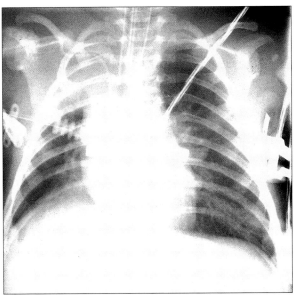

Fig. 313 Unexplained hypoxia was clarified by the chest radiograph. The tracheal tube is too long, and has entered the left main bronchus. The right lung has collapsed as a result. Withdrawal of the tracheal tube should ensure re-expansion.

OBSTRUCTION OF THE MAIN BRONCHUS CAUSING COLLAPSE

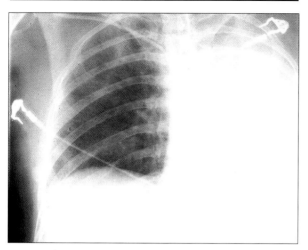

Fig. 314 The upper main bronchus is occluded by the tracheal tube.

COLLAPSED RIGHT UPPER LOBE

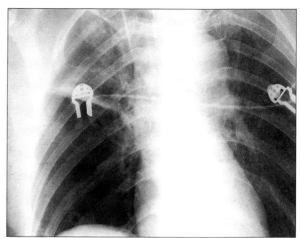

Fig. 315 Collapsed right upper lobe.

PLUG IN LEFT MAIN BRONCHUS

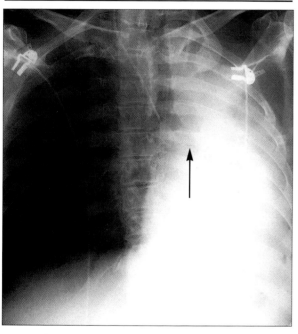

Fig. 316 Note the absence of an air bronchogram and the way the left main bronchus suddenly stops (arrow). This indicates a plug of mucus is present.

TENTING OF DIAPHRAGM

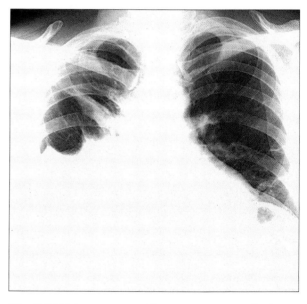

Fig. 317 This suggests a fibrotic process in the lung.

LATERAL FILM SHOWING TENTING OF DIAPHRAGM

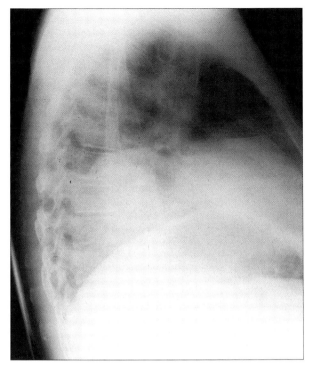

Fig. 318 Lateral film showing tenting of diaphragm.

ULTRASOUND OF ABSCESS

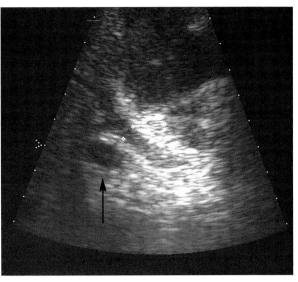

Fig. 319 This shows an abscess cavity at the bed of the gallbladder (arrow).

ULTRASOUND OF ASCITES

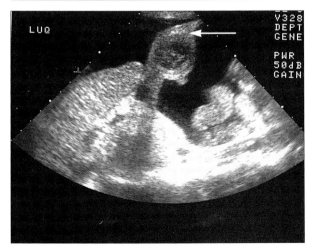

Fig. 320 The bowel (arrow) can be seen surrounded by ascitic fluid.

ULTRASOUND OF HAEMOTHORAX

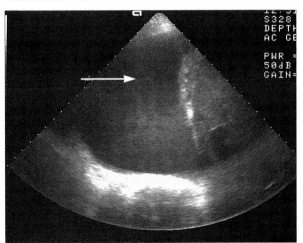

Fig. 321 A large haemothorax is demonstrated (arrow), secondary to attempted subclavian line insertion.

Chapter 4 **Cardiology in the ICU**

HYPERTENSION

The World Health Organisation (WHO) definition of hypertension is a blood pressure exceeding 160/95 mmHg. The incidence increases with age. In only about 1% of the population screened can a specific cause be found. Secondary hypertension may result from renal disease, pregnancy, pain, endocrine and vascular disorders and some medication, e.g. contraceptive pill. Hypertension is associated with obesity and alcoholism.

HYPERTENSIVE RETINOPATHY

Fig. 322 The vessels show increasing tortuosity, flame-shaped retinal haemorrhages and soft 'cotton wool' exudates. The fundii of all critically ill patients should be examined, as they can give valuable pre-existing information about disease in the patient.

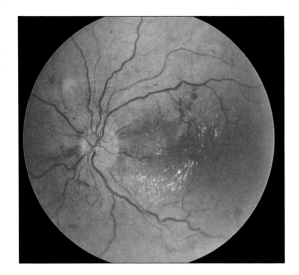

LEFT VENTRICULAR HYPERTROPHY (LVH)

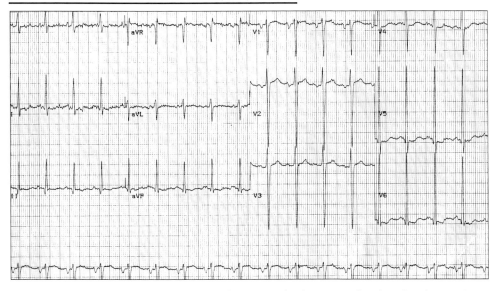

Fig. 323 Hypertension may lead to left ventricular hypertrophy (LVH). The ECG in hypertension may show severe signs of LVH: the amplitude of the trace is halved. The R wave in V5 and V6 and the S wave in V1 and V2 together exceed 45 mm. There is also T-wave inversion.

POSTOPERATIVE HYPERTENSION

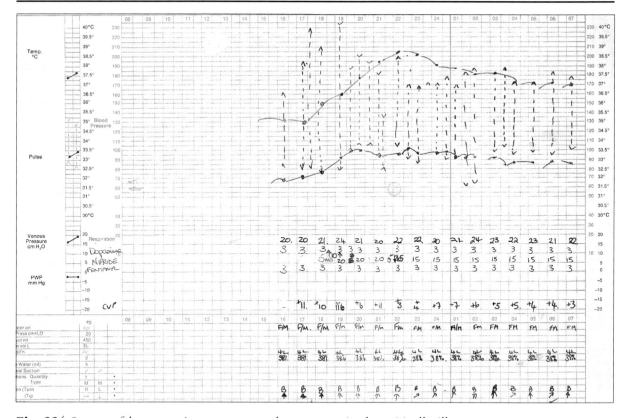

Fig. 324 Surges of hypertension are extremely common in the critically ill patient after vascular and cardiac surgery. In this case a peak of 230 mmHg was reached. Adequate analgesia and sedation (with morphine, propofol or midalozam) may help. Failing that, specific antihypertensive treatment, such as nifedipine or a nitrate infusion, can be used.

UNCOMMON CAUSES OF HYPERTENSION

Table 15 Causes of secondary hypertension

Disease	
Renal	Glomerulonephritis
	Pyelonephritis
	Polycystic kidneys
	Analgesic nephropathy
	Renal artery stenosis
Cardiac	Coarction of the aorta
Pregnancy	Toxaemia
Endocrine	Cushing's disease
	Phaeochromocytoma
	Conn's syndrome
	Hyperparathyroidism
	Acromegaly
Drugs	Oral contraceptives
	Corticosteroids
	Monoamine oxidase inhibitors

RENAL ARTERY STENOSIS

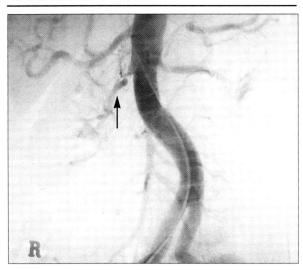

Fig. 325 There is a severe stenosis of the left renal artery (arrow) leading to hypertension.

PHAEOCHROMOCYTOMA

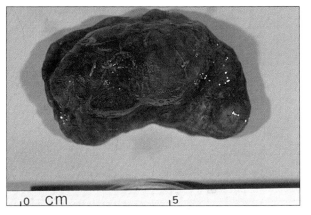

Fig. 326 Caused by a rare tumour-secreting catecholamine arising from the adrenal gland or along the sympathetic chain, phaeochromocytoma can be multiple and the symptoms mistaken for pre-eclampsia in pregnancy.

COARCTATION OF THE AORTA

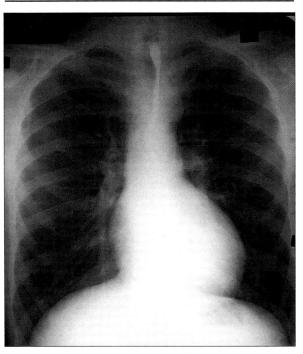

Fig. 327 There is notching of the ribs. The aorta shows a characteristic 'dumbbell' shadow where the coarctation occurs.

OBSTRUCTIVE SHOCK

In this form of shock a decreasing cardiac output is caused by a reduction in venous return. There are many causes for this, including pneumothorax, PEEP or pulmonary embolism or actual restriction of the heart size, e.g. pericardial effusion, tamponade.

PERICARDIAL TAMPONADE

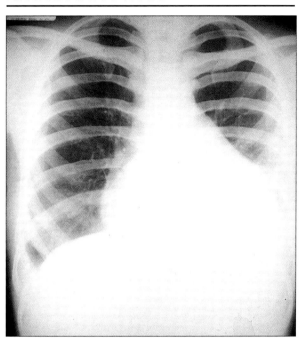

Fig. 328 This chest radiograph shows the classical enlargement of the pericardium up to the root of the aorta obliterating the aortic notch. The rapid accumulation of fluid within the pericardium (tamponade) will dramatically reduce the venous return and lead to death if untreated.

PULMONARY EMBOLISM

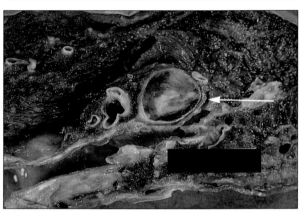

Fig. 329 This is a massive pulmonary embolism (arrow). Death was immediate. Arising in the deep veins above the knee in 95% of cases (see **Fig. 32**, p. 12).

POSITIVE END EXPIRATORY PRESSURE (PEEP)

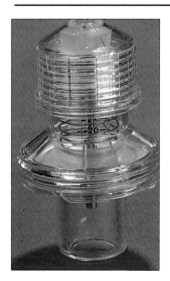

Fig. 330 Positive end expiratory pressure (PEEP) is the term used when pressure is applied at the end of exhalation in the intubated, ventilated patient. Ignoring how this is achieved, the result is an increase in FRC because of alveolar recruitment. The price that is paid, especially in hypovolaemic patients, may be a reduction in cardiac output by decreasing venous return. The other harmful effect is to increase intrathoracic pressure that may result in a pneumothorax, particularly if the patient strains against the tracheal tube. Small values of 5–10 cmH$_2$O are usually well tolerated.

V/Q SCAN OF PULMONARY EMBOLISM

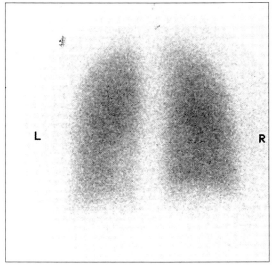
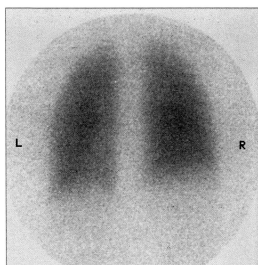
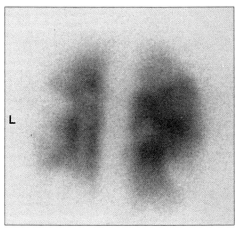
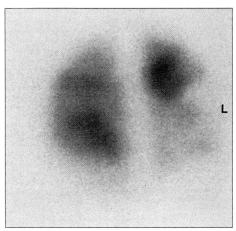

Figs 331–334 The perfusion scans shows large defects that are not perfused, which is consistent with multiple emboli. Ventilation inhalation (**331**, top left); ventilation equilibrium (**332**, top right); posterior perfusion (**333**, bottom left); and anterior perfusion (**334**, bottom right). Although this is the most useful diagnostic test for pulmonary embolism, it has limitations.

CARDIAC OUTPUT

Measurement of cardiac output is now an integral part of management of shock. A thermodilution pulmonary artery catheter (PAC) (see **Fig. 382**, p. 112) carries a thermistor 4 cm from the catheter tip.

By injecting 10 ml of ice cold saline into the right atrium a 'cooling' curve can be drawn, from which the cardiac output can be computed.

THERMODILUTION EQUIPMENT

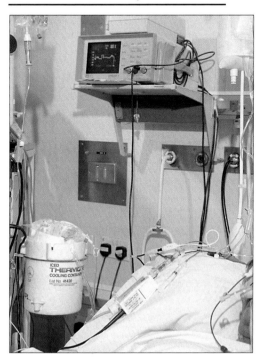

Fig. 335 Seen here are the ice bucket, the PAC *in situ* and the cardiac output computer on a shelf above. This system uses an oximetric PAC requiring a separate monitor. There are also cardiac output modules for most monitors to integrate with existing systems.

Table 16 Normal values in haemodynamic monitoring

Site	Pressure (mmHg)	Mean
Right atrium	0–5	
Right ventricle	30–15/5–0	
Pulmonary artery	30–15/12–4	9–16
Pulmonary wedge	6-12	

Flows		Units
Cardiac output	4–8	l/min
Cardiac index	2.8–4.2	$l/min/m^2$

PRINT-OUT OF 'COOLING' CURVE

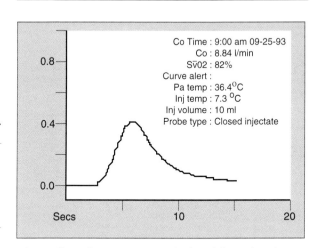

Fig. 336 Cardiac output is calculated from the change in temperature of blood as it flows past the tip of the catheter. The value for cardiac output may be less accurate as the injectate temperature has risen above 0°C. It should be repeated at the correct temperature, otherwise the results are misleading.

ECHOCARDIOGRAM

ECHOCARDIOGRAPHY: LEFT VENTRICULAR HYPERTROPHY

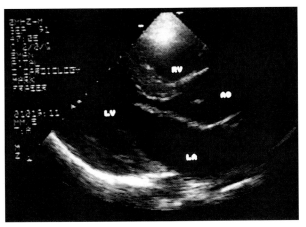

Fig. 337 The normal chambers of the heart displayed on an echocardiogram.

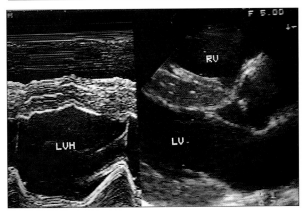

Fig. 338 The most useful bedside test after ECG is echocardiography, which can also be performed by the oesophageal route (see **Fig. 353**, p. 103). This test will provide valuable information on flow dynamics and detect effusions, tamponade, valvular, congenital and heart abnormalities.

ISCHAEMIC HEART DISEASE/INFARCTION

Coronary heart disease is the commonest cause of death in the Western hemisphere. The condition often presents as angina, caused by at least a 50% reduction in coronary artery blood flow. If a decent collateral circulation is absent, angina may be precipitated by exercise, cold weather, or emotion leading to ischaemia of the ventricle.

The sudden occlusion of a main coronary artery, usually caused by a thrombosis, results in infarction. This is often a retrospective diagnosis in the critically ill based on ECG and enzyme changes. Many patients have 'silent' infarcts as a result of their illness that lack the clinical features of chest pain, pallor, sweating and nausea.

ECG: ISCHAEMIA

Fig. 339 The trace shows the characteristic ST wave inversion in V4–6. If the ECG changes transiently to these ischaemic patterns, nitrates are helpful in reversing the trend.

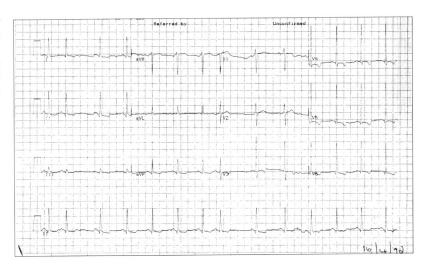

ECG: ANTERIOR MYOCARDIAL INFARCT

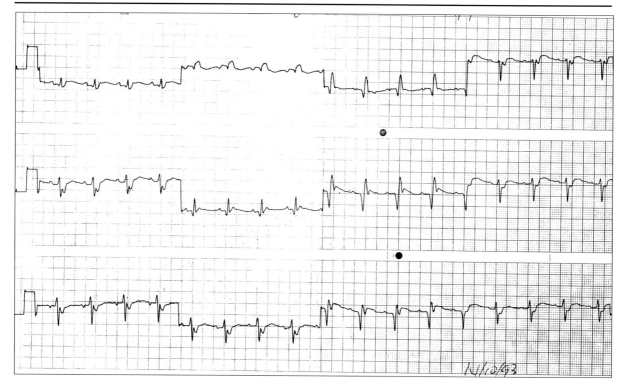

Fig. 340 A pathological Q wave is seen in V1–V5. There is ST segment elevation in V2–V6. Reciprocal changes (ST depression) leads II, III and aVF.

HISTOLOGY OF MYOCARDIAL INFARCT

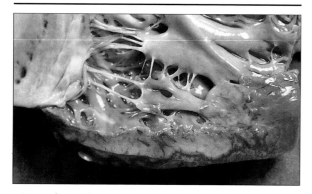

Fig. 341 Pale area of acute infarction in the myocardium.

ECG: INFERIOR MYOCARDIAL INFARCT

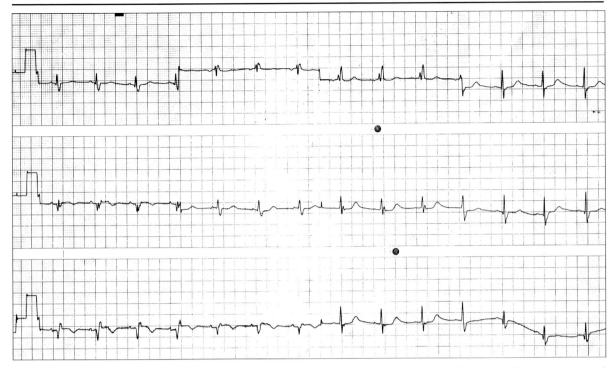

Fig. 342 Pathological Q waves are seen: II, III and aVF. ST segment elevation in leads II, III and aVF. Reciprocal changes V1–V6, 1 and aVL.

CREATINE KINASE-MB

Table 17 Creatine kinase-MB

Clinical details	Specimen type: serum
Chest pain	
CK-MB concentration	105 μg/l

(CK-MB mass:peak values >6.5 at 12–24 h is consistent with MI)

These results are diagnostic of myocardial infarct. The isoenzyme is principally found in the cardiac muscle.

Some laboratories measure CK-MB differently, and report the results as unit/l. Most accept a significant result as being in excess of 25 units/l with this value being 6–30% of the total CK value.

ENZYME ACTIVITY AND MYOCARDIAL INFARCT

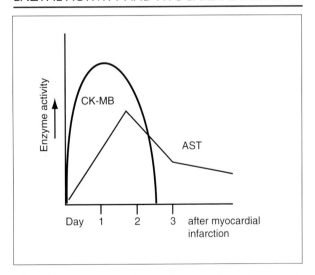

Fig. 343 Increase of the the creatine kinase-MB isoenzyme is now considered diagnostic, but because of the rapid increase and decrease of CK-MB serial enzyme samples at 12-hour periods are required. Aspartate aminotransferase (AST) is also increased, but at a later phase.

THALLIUM SCAN

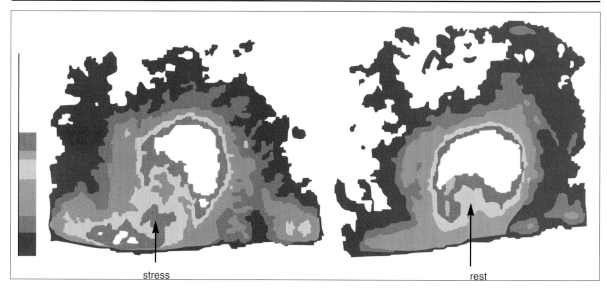

stress   rest

Fig. 344 A radioisotope study of the left ventricle demonstrating a large fixed inferior defect, consistent with an infarct. The septum (left) shows some recirculation consistent with ischaemia. Radioisotope studies are helpful in confirming the diagnosis of myocardial infarction when enzyme tests are equivocal.

CHEST RADIOGRAPH: 'BATWING' PULMONARY OEDEMA

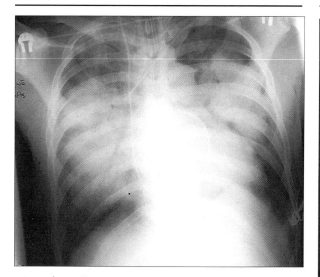

Fig. 345 A florid example of severe left ventricular failure leading to pulmonary oedema after myocardial infarction. Oxygen, diuretics, ventilation and PEEP are used in the treatment. A PAC permits differentiation of ARDS with a normal wedge pressure. The PAC should not be inserted during extreme hypoxia.

PULMONARY OEDEMA FLUID

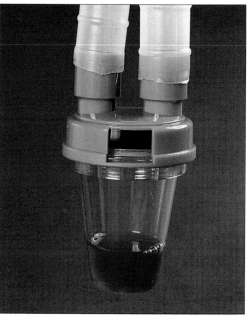

Fig. 346 This brown fluid pours up the airway and will asphyxiate the patient unless the situation is reversed.

ECG: HEART BLOCK

Fig. 347 Complete heart block. Heart block occurring with an inferior infarct tends to be transient , with an anterior infarct permanent. A pacemaker is required.

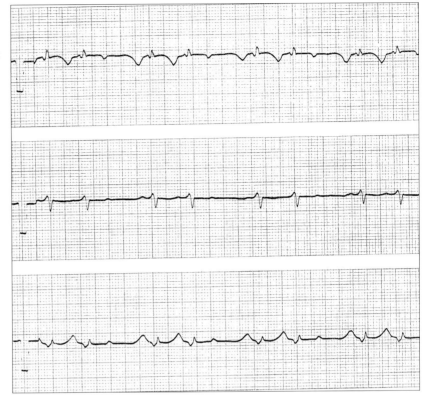

PACEMAKER

Fig. 348 The pacing wire is positioned in contact with the right ventricle. The use of a pacing wire is not just used in heart block: it can also be helpful in low output states.

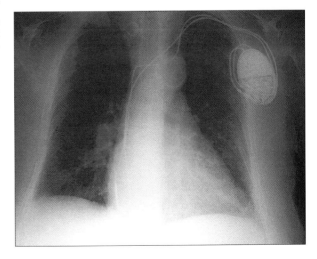

ECG: PACED HEART BLOCK

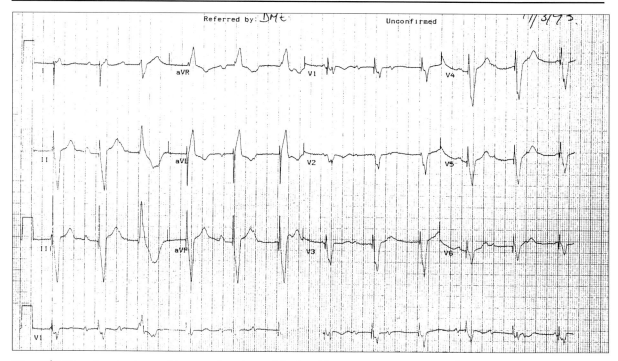

Fig. 349 Here is a patient with complete heart block with a permanent pacemaker *in situ.*

HEART FAILURE/INFECTIONS OF THE HEART

MYOCARDITIS: CHEST RADIOGRAPH OF PULMONARY OEDEMA

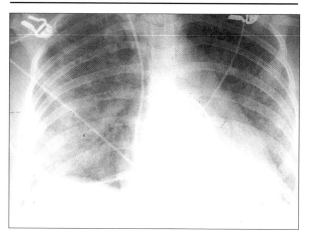

Fig. 350 A 23-year-old primigravida with severe eclampsia delivered a stillborn child. She developed fulminating pulmonary oedema. Her wedge pressure was 30 mmHg, her PAP was 40/30 mmHg (see **Table 16**, p. 96 for normal values) and her systemic blood pressure 200/90 mmHg. On 60% oxygen with 10 cm of PEEP she maintained a PaO$_2$ of 8.5 (saturation 90%). She required 14 days of diuretics, vasodilator therapy and ventilation to reverse this situation. A herpes simplex myocarditis was responsible.

CONGESTIVE HEART FAILURE: BILATERAL LEG OEDEMA

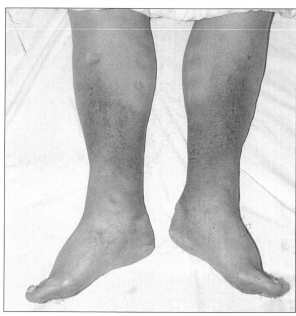

Fig. 351 Patients with long-standing heart failure develop bilateral pitting oedema.

SEPTIC EMBOLI

Fig. 352 Embolic infarcts from the heart. Repeated episodes of infection especially after invasive monitoring, in drug addicts and patients with prosthetic valves should raise the question of this diagnosis.

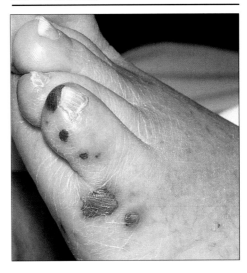

TRANSOESOPHAGEAL ECHOCARDIOGRAPHY

Fig. 353 The best view of the mitral and aortic valves is using transoesophageal echocardiography; even so, the diagnosis can be elusive. Here is a view showing a large vegetation on the mitral valve (arrow).

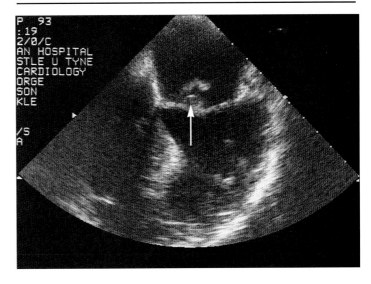

PATHOLOGY OF BACTERIAL ENDOCARDITIS

Fig. 354 The valve has numerous vegetations. Treatment is surgical replacement of the valve with prolonged high dose antibiotic cover.

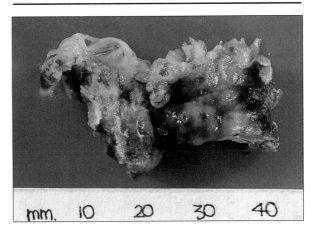

RESUSCITATION

The training of individuals in cardiopulmonary resuscitation is an essential feature of clinical practice. These skills need to be rehearsed and reinforced every six months to ensure competence in staff not meeting cardiac arrest often. Every branch of hospital personnel should attend these courses.

TRAINING MANNEQUIN

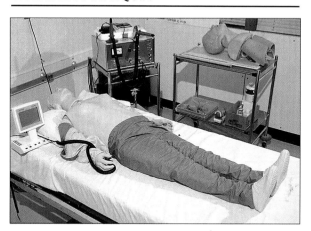

Fig. 355 A training room allows small numbers to practise their skills with expert tuition to hand.

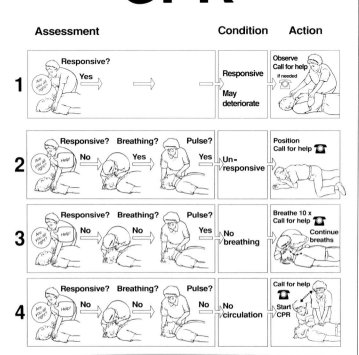

Fig. 356 CPR Emergency Action Plan. The steps in CPR are set out based on European guidelines so everyone can understand what is to be done, in what order and why.

NOTE: The American Heart Association (standards and guidelines, 1986) makes different recommendations from the European standard drug dosages quoted:
  Epinephrine (adrenaline) iv 0.5 mg and repeat at 5 min intervals.
  Atropine iv 0.5 mg and repeat at 5 min intervals, up to 2 mg maximum.
  Sodium bicarbonate is no longer recommended for routine administering. If used, sodium bicarbonate iv 8.4% 1 meq/kg.

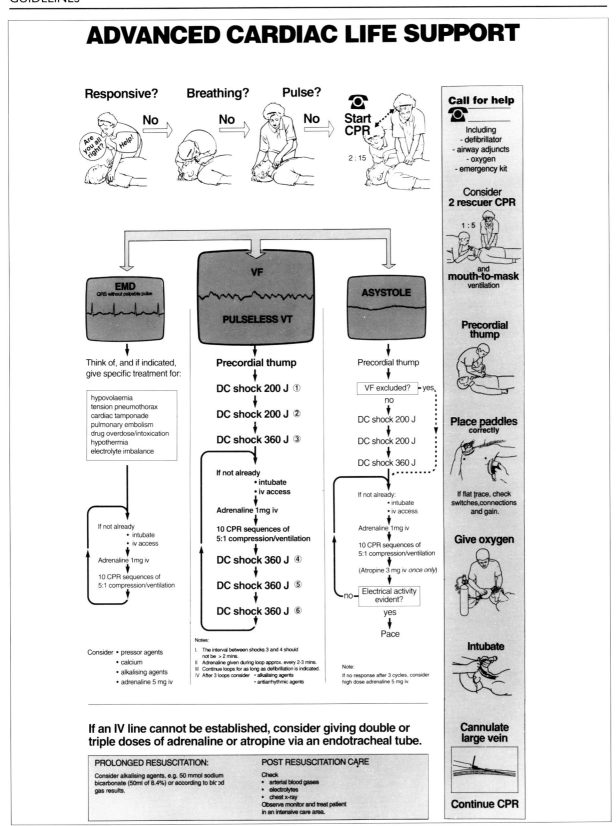

Fig. 357 Advanced cardiac life support.

WARD EDUCATION

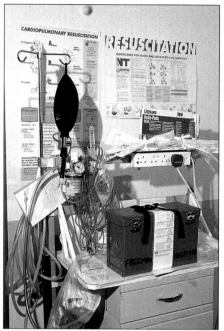

Fig. 358 All wards should carry detailed guidance on how to resuscitate in an easy to follow manner. The equipment needs to be at hand.

DRUGS

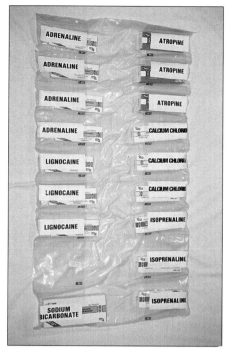

Fig. 359 The drugs are best provided premixed and in syringes to be given immediately.

DISORDERS OF RHYTHM

Dysrhythmias are common in ill patients, and with a little experience most can be easily recognised. Abnormal heart rhythms are often classified according to their effect on heart rate. The causes are not always clear, though hypoxia, sepsis, electrolyte disturbances and a silent MI are common causes in the critically ill.

REGULAR FAST HEART RATES

SINUS TACHYCARDIA

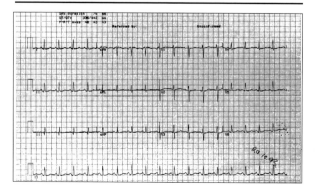

Fig. 360 A regular fast heart rate, between 100 and 180 beats/min. Each beat is preceded by a P wave. The common causes are fear, pain, exercise, stimulant drugs (atropine, isoprenaline), fever, anaemia and shock.

VENTRICULAR TACHYCARDIA

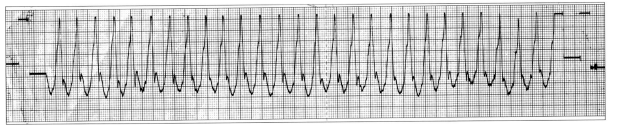

Fig. 361 A serious life threatening arrhythmia, with a rate between 150 and 200 beats/min. A common cause of sudden death. Lignocaine may stop it.

SUPRAVENTRICULAR TACHYCARDIA

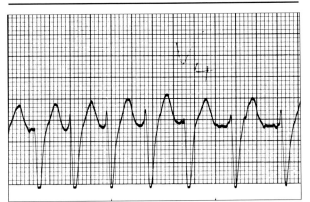

Fig. 362 Created by an atrial ectopic focus or at the arteriovenous junction and are paroxysmal in nature, (therefore described as paroxysmal atrial tachycardia and paroxysmal nodal tachycardia, respectively) and often precipitated by coffee or alcohol in the normal heart. Pain, anxiety, tracheal suction or hypoxia may start it in the seriously ill.

ATRIAL FLUTTER: REGULAR VENTRICULAR RESPONSE

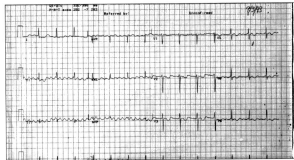

Fig. 363 The characteristic 'saw-tooth' appearance makes this diagnosis unmistakable. A flutter rate of 200–350 beats/min is seen. Always associated with underlying heart disease.

SLOW REGULAR RHYTHM

SINUS BRADYCARDIA

Fig. 364 A slow regular rate under 60 beats/min. Common in all age groups and associated with trained athletes. Seen medically in association with drugs (e.g. digoxin, ß blockade), myocardial infarction and anaesthesia.

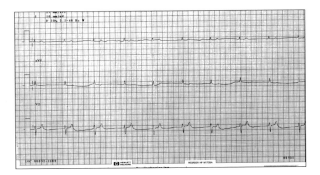

IRREGULAR PULSE RATES

ECTOPIC BEATS

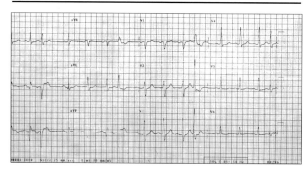

Fig. 365 This ECG shows multifocal ventricular ectopic beats. Isolated ectopic beats are common and do not require treatment. If showers occur then they may precede more serious arrhythmias. Associated with ischaemia, MI, drugs (digoxin) and hyperkalaemia.

BIGEMINY

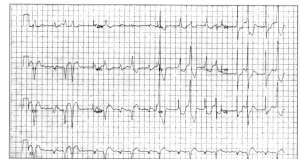

Fig. 366 A nodal induced beat (with inverted P wave) is followed by a ventricular extrasystole.

ATRIAL FIBRILLATION

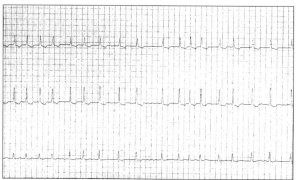

Fig. 367 The P waves are absent, and an irregular fibrillation wave at a rate of 400–600 beats/min with an irregular heart rate of 140–170 beats/min. This is one of the most common arrhythmias seen in the critically ill.

VENTRICULAR FIBRILLATION

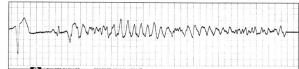

Fig. 368 A rapid, chaotic rhythm of ineffective ventricular contraction. Death will follow if the patient is not defibrillated.

SOME OTHER ECG DISTURBANCES

PERICARDITIS AND MYOCARDITIS

Fig. 369 The changes show ST elevation in all leads. The CK-MB was increased, at 8 μg/l (normal <6.5 μg/l). This 32-year-old man presented in extremis with acute left ventricular failure and an ejection fraction of 19% after a flu-like illness.

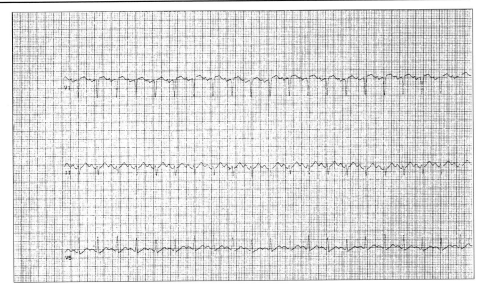

DIGOXIN TOXICITY

Fig. 370 The characteristic inverted tick seen in the ST segment is shown in this example.

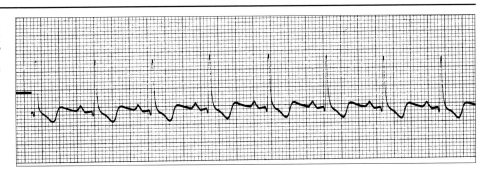

HYPERKALAEMIA

Fig. 371 QRS widening, high peaked T-wave indicating a near lethal situation are shown in this example of hyperkalaemia.

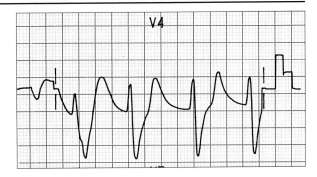

MONITORING

The use of invasive monitoring techniques is established practice in ICU. The insertion of such lines requires skill and knowledge, and is not without harmful complications.

It is therefore important that staff are familiar with the use of transducer systems: the fact that they must be zeroed to provide reliable information each time the patient is monitored. If their position in relation to the patient's body is not changed, the values they give will be wrong. This increases the dangers posed by monitoring. Air bubbles in the transducer are a common cause of a damped and inaccurate trace.

ARTERIAL CUT DOWN

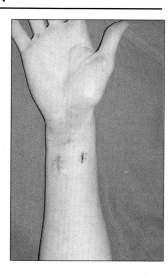

Fig. 372 In situations where percutaneous insertion of arterial lines prove impossible an arterial line can be inserted under direct vision. This is most unusual today.

BLACK PATCH I

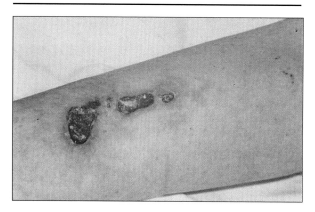

Fig. 373 Thrombosis of the radial artery is common, but only infrequently does it result in infarction of the skin or fingers.

BLACK PATCH 2

Fig. 374 The radial artery is most commonly chosen because of a collateral circulation from the ulnar artery. A 20 gauge parallel sided cannula with a continuous heparin flush is preferred.

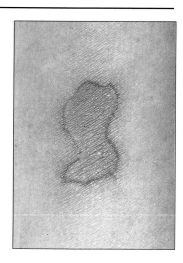

COMPLICATIONS

Table 18 Complications of arterial lines

Common	Less frequent	Rare
Failure	Ischaemia	Necrotic skin
Pain	Embolism	Drug mistake
Bruising	Bleeding	Aneurysm
Infection		A–V fistula
Thrombosis		Limb necrosis

Pain and bruising are common. The arterial line is best nursed visibly to witness any disconnection or leak, usually after sampling, and marked to avoid drug injection.

INTRA-ARTERIAL PHENYTOIN

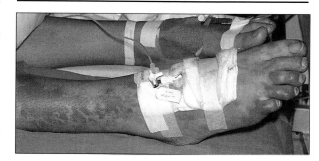

Fig. 375 A nurse has given the drug into the arterial line in the mistaken belief this was the correct route. The foot is necrotic. The dorsalis pedis artery is the next most popular site for an arterial line.

CENTRAL VEIN ACCESS

The majority of admissions to a general ICU will require a central venous line to measure CVP, infuse drugs and permit feeding. Special lines are used to undertake dialysis and to use a rapid infusion system.

The principal difficulties are insertion failure, arterial puncture and pneumothorax. The subclavian route has an unenviable reputation for serious complications, but no route is without limitations.

Table 19 Complications of central venous catheters

General	Specific problems	Rare
Infection	Arterial puncture	Nerve injury
Thrombosis	Pneumo/haemothorax	Tracheal injury
Phlebitis	Air embolism	Chylothorax
Failure	Ectopic infusion	Myocardial perforation
	Vein perforation	Arrhythmia
	Endocarditis	Breakage
	Tangled lines	Horner's syndrome
	Arrhythmias	Arterio-venous fistula
		Death

SPAGHETTI JUNCTION

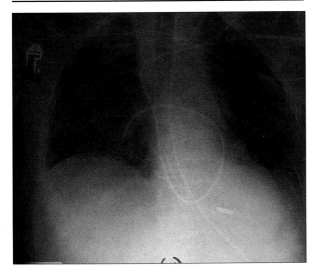

Fig. 376 The number of access lines can make radiograph interpretation very confusing. From right to left this patient has horizontal ECG leads, a rapid infusion system in the right internal jugular, a tracheal tube, a nasogastric tube, a gastroenterostomy tube, a left internal jugular central line, and a left subclavian pulmonary artery catheter (which is in too far).

Fig. 378 A combination of low platelets and an arterial puncture resulted in this haematoma during attempted central venous cannulation. Pressure for over 30 min was required to stop the bleeding. About 1% of all attempts results in arterial puncture.

CENTRAL LINE INDUCED PNEUMOTHORAX

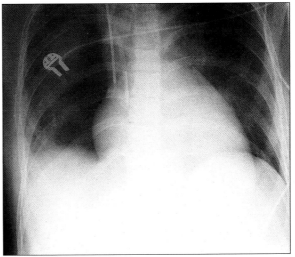

Fig. 377 Pneumothorax occurs in 1–2% of all attempts. A chest radiograph is mandatory after insertion.

SEVERE BRUISING

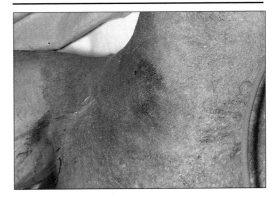

VEIN DAMAGE

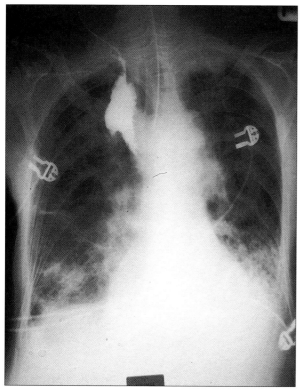

Fig. 379 This apparently successful right internal jugular line has damaged the superior vena cava.

CRYSTALLOID EFFUSION

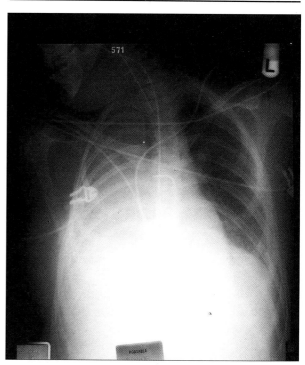

Fig. 380 A left subclavian line insertion has damaged the right pleura, resulting in the infusion fluid collecting in the right pleural cavity.

TANGLED LINE

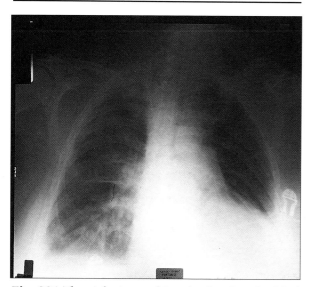

Fig. 381 The right internal jugular line has doubled back on itself. Radiograph screening and care is needed to remove this and leave the patient unharmed.

PULMONARY ARTERY CATHETER (PAC)

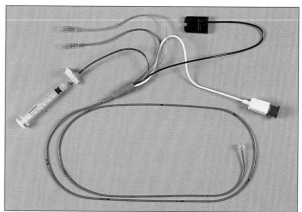

Fig. 382 The modern PAC can combine a number of functions. This is a fibreoptic pulmonary catheter providing a continuous venous saturation (see **Fig. 209**, p. 60). Pulmonary artery and central venous pressure can be continuously measured. Cardiac output (red cap) can be achieved by thermodilution and a 'wedge' pressure obtained by inflating the balloon and letting the catheter float from its location in the pulmonary artery to temporarily occlude a distal vessel (see **Fig. 383**, p. 113). Not shown here is a pacing facility.

Table 20 Complications of PAC usage

Insertion	*In situ*	Technical
Arrhythmias	Migration	Damping
Coiling/loops	Balloon rupture	Motion artifact
Knots	Bacterial endocarditis	Malposition
Valvular damage	Fragmentation	Loss of trace
Incorrect site	Pulmonary infarction	
Vessel damage	Arrhythmia	
	Haemorrhage	
	Decrease in platelet numbers	

Fig. 383 The pressure wave changes from a pulmonary artery (PA) trace to the flatter pulmonary 'wedge' (PCW) or the occlusion position is a distal small pulmonary artery. Transient arrhythmias are common on insertion. This procedure should not be attempted in severely ill patients until their airways are secure and they are not hypoxic.

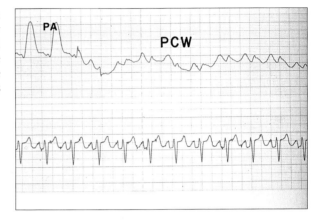

KNOT IN CATHETER

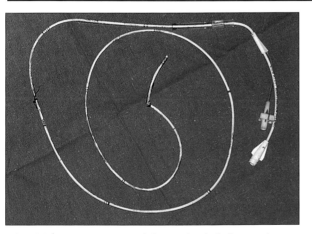

Fig. 384 A PAC inserted from the left femoral vein coiled in the heart.

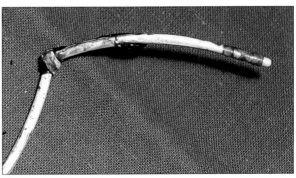

Fig. 385 A single throw knot occurred when the catheter became tangled.

MECHANICAL ASSIST DEVICES

INTRA-AORTIC BALLOON PUMP

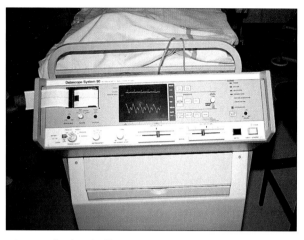

Fig. 386 The balloon is inserted via the femoral artery. Inflation of the balloon, placed just below the aortic arch, is synchronised to coincide with the end of systole. Then, blood is directed in a retrograde manner to improve coronary artery and aortic arch perfusion, instead of going further down the aorta. The balloon deflates during diastole. This technique is useful in low output states.

EXTRACORPOREAL MEMBRANE OXYGENATION (ECMO)

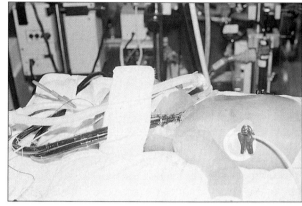

Fig. 387 A venous-arterial device to improve poor gas exchange. In this patient venous access is from the right internal jugular vein and returns through the right common carotid artery.

ECMO OXYGENATOR

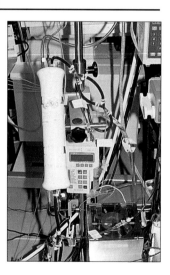

Fig. 388 Continuous heparinisation and supervision is needed. Technically complicated but with good results to date, especially in neonates and children.

INTRAVENOUS OXYGENATOR (IVOX)

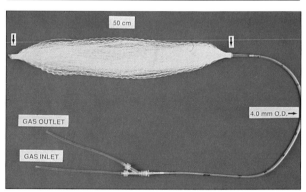

Fig. 389 This mesh is unfurled in the inferior vena cava after surgical insertion. Simpler than ECMO (see **Fig. 388** adjacent), it works by providing enhanced venous oxygenation. The method is still undergoing evaluation.

Chapter 5 **The role of the laboratory**

BLOOD GASES

The analysis of arterial blood gases provides quick and reproducible information on how efficiently the lungs and kidneys are working. The data provided are pH or (H^+), PaO_2, $PaCO_2$, and derived bicarbonate and oxygen saturation. Normal values are shown in **Table 21**.

Table 21 Arterial blood gases

		or	
pH	7.36–7.44	or	(H^+) 36–44 nmol/l
PaO_2	11–14 kPa		83–105 mmHg
$PaCO_2$	4.6–6.0 kPa		35–45 mmHg
Bicarbonate	22–28 mmol/l		
Saturation	>95%		

MEASUREMENT OF ARTERIAL BLOOD GAS

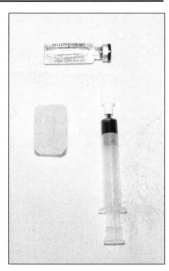

Fig. 390 There are three basic components for successful sampling: a heparinised syringe, a well-mixed arterial sample (without air bubbles), and storage on ice if a blood gas machine is not immediately available.

BLOOD GAS MACHINE

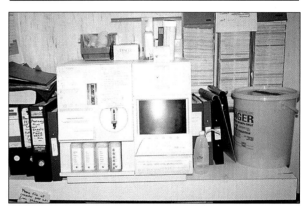

Fig. 391 This is a sophisticated analyser that requires regular quality control at least twice a day. A co-oximeter is advisable when measuring oxygen saturation, since it is more accurate when measuring saturation. All staff using the machine need instruction to ensure consistent and safe usage. Breakdowns are expensive and deny patients the benefits of rapid blood gas analysis.

HENDERSON EQUATION

The relationship of respiratory and renal function is expressed in the Henderson equation:

(H^+) (nmol/l) = Constant $\times$ $PaCO_2$/Bicarbonate

Fig. 392 Respiratory compensation is a rapid way to cope with acid–base disturbances; in the longer term, renal function determines new bicarbonate formation and acid excretion.

HENDERSON–HASSELBALCH EQUATION

$$pH = pKa + \log_{10}\frac{(HCO_3^-)}{(H_2CO_3)}$$

pKa = Dissociation constant
(pH at which 50% of a base or acid is ionised)

Fig. 393 Buffers are capable of maintaining the pH of a given solution by dissociation to produce a weak acid with a conjugate base or vice versa.

Table 22 Metabolic acid–base disturbances

Metabolic acidosis	Metabolic alkalosis
mechanism	
Loss of bicarbonate or addition of acid	Loss of acid or addition of alkali
causes	
Renal failure	Vomiting
Diabetic coma	Nasogastric suction
Starvation	Diuretics
Shock	
Diarrhoea	**intake/ingestion**
Fistula	Bicarbonate
Renal tubular acidosis	
intake/ingestion	**mineralocorticoid**
Ethyl alcohol	Hyperaldosteronism
Methyl alcohol	Cushing's disease
NH_4Cl	

METABOLIC ACIDOSIS: CHRONIC RENAL FAILURE

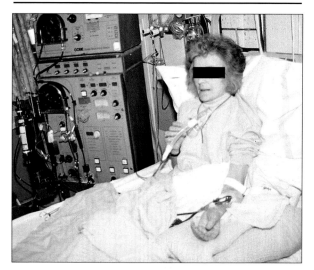

Fig. 394 Dialysis is required three times a week to maintain this patient in a stable situation. Blood gases:
pH = 7.32 (H^+ = 48 nmol/l)
$PaCO_2$ = 3.5 kPa
bicarbonate = 16 mmol/l.

METABOLIC ALKALOSIS: EXCESSIVE GASTRIC LOSSES

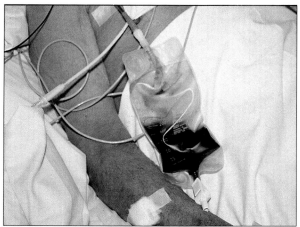

Fig. 395 Gastric ileus. Blood gases:
pH = 7.6 (H^+ = 25 nmol/l)
$PaCO_2$ = 5.3 kPa
bicarbonate = 38 mmol/l.

Table 23 Illustrative changes in metabolic alkalosis and acidosis

	H^+ (nmol/l)	pH	$PaCO_2$ (kPa)	Plasma bicarbonate (mmol/l)
Normal range	36–44	7.36–7.44	4.6–6.0	22–28
Condition				
Metabolic alkalosis				
Acute	25	7.60	5.3	38
With respiratory compensation	30	7.52	6.6	40
Metabolic acidosis				
Acute	90	7.05	5.3	11
With partial respiratory compensation	76	7.12	3.2	8

Table 24 Some causes of respiratory disturbances

Respiratory acidosis	Respiratory alkalosis
mechanism	
Hypoventilation $PaCO_2 > 7$ kPA	Hypoventilation $PaCO_2 < 3.2$ kPA
causes	
Central drive depression	Anxiety/hysteria
Trauma	Pain
Drug overdose	Excessive mechanical ventilation
Obesity	Shock
Infection	Hypoxia
Brain tumour	Sepsis
	Altitude
Neuromuscular	Fibrosis
Polio	Drugs, e.g. salicylates
Guillain–Barré	Central disorders
Myasthenia	
Electrolytes, e.g. low K^+	
Chest wall	
Crushed chest	
Kyphoscoliosis	
Intrinsic lung disease	
COPD	
Pneumonia	
Oedema	
Fibrosis	
Airway obstruction	
Tumour	
Epiglottitis	

RESPIRATORY ACIDOSIS: HEAD INJURY

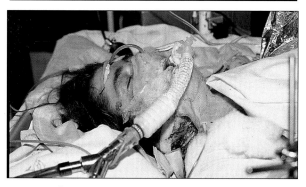

Fig. 396 A well-recognised cause of primary respiratory depression.
pH = 7.30 (H$^+$ = 50 nmol/l)
PaCO$_2$ = 7.6 kPa
bicarbonate = 28 mmol/l.

RESPIRATORY ALKALOSIS: ALTITUDE

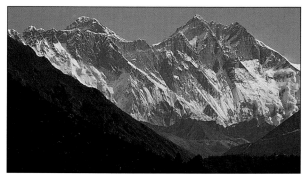

Fig. 397 Mount Everest, altitude 8,848 m. Blood gases from a simulated ascent of Everest were measured as:
pH = 7.56 (H$^+$ = 28 nmol/l)
PaCO$_2$ = 1.5
PaO$_2$ = 4 kPa.

ALTITUDE PULMONARY OEDEMA

Fig. 398 A stricken mountaineer with pulmonary oedema being treated inside a portable pressure chamber (Gamow Bag) at Pheriche, a village near Mount Everest, altitude 4300 m. Air is pumped under pressure by a foot pump. Such intervention can be life saving.

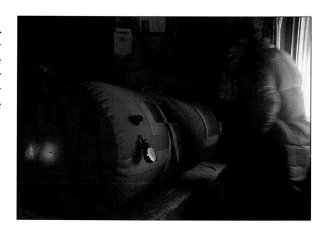

Table 25 Illustrative changes in respiratory acidosis and alkalosis in patients with normal lungs and with chronic obstructive pulmonary disease (COPD)

	H$^+$ (nmol/l)	pH	PaCO$_2$ (kPa)	Plasma bicarbonate (mmol/l)
Normal range	36–44	7.36–7.44	4.6–6.0	22–28
Condition				
Respiratory acidosis				
acute (normal lungs)	50	7.30	10	36
metabolic compensation	45	7.35	10	41
acute COPD	55	7.26	8.5	28
compensation	45	7.35	7.8	32
Respiratory alkalosis				
acute	30	7.52	3.2	19
metabolic compensation	36	7.44	3.6	18

OXYGENATION

The goal of all treatment is to achieve sufficient arterial oxygenation to maintain an oxygen saturation >90%. Monitoring with an oximeter is helpful.

Table 26 Oxygenation: normal values

Arterial tension	11–14 kPa	83–105 mmHg
Arterial content	8.9–9.4 kPa	20–21 vol%
Arterial saturation	95%	

ANOXIC ANOXIA

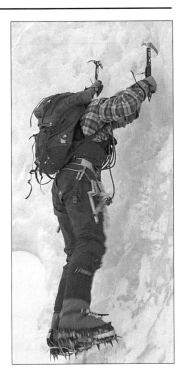

Fig. 399 Altitude, house fires, and right-to-left shunts are examples of this condition.

ANAEMIC ANOXIA

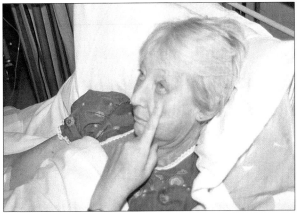

Fig. 400 Insufficient haemoglobin to carry oxygen to the tissues. A haemoglobin of 10 g/dl is considered acceptable in acute situations.

STAGNANT ANOXIA

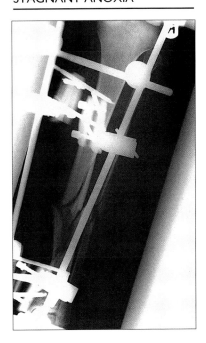

Fig. 401 Poor circulation after injury results in fully oxygenated blood flowing slowly through the periphery having a large quantity of oxygen extracted.

HISTOTOXIC ANOXIA: CARBON MONOXIDE POISONING

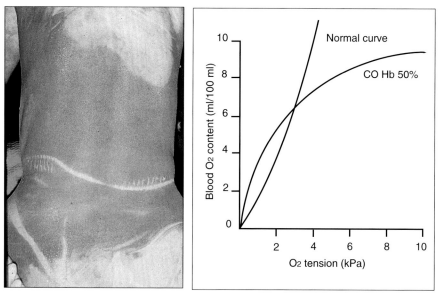

Figs 402 and **403** Carboxyhaemoglobin results in poor oxygen binding to haemoglobin as carbon monoxide has an affinity for haemoglobin 240 times greater than oxygen.

NUTRITION

Adequate nutrition is fundamental for survival. Assessment includes weight, plasma albumin concentration and leucocyte count. Failure to feed results in increased rates of sepsis and a higher mortality.

NUTRITIONAL OEDEMA

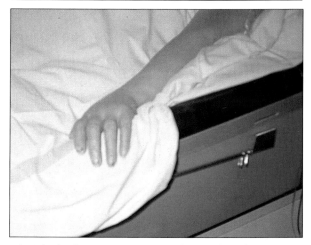

Fig. 404 This patient was admitted with massive oedema affecting the whole body and albumin of 18 g/l. Serial serum albumin remains the reference value for adequacy of nutrition.

24-HOUR URINE

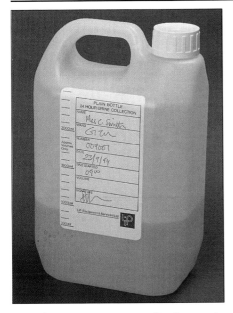

Fig. 405 Measurement of urinary nitrogen (80% of total daily excretion) from this sample allows a reasonable estimate of total daily nitrogen losses, thus allowing sensible nutritional replacement. The urinary nitrogen loss was 18.7 g/24 hours.

BOWEL FISTULA

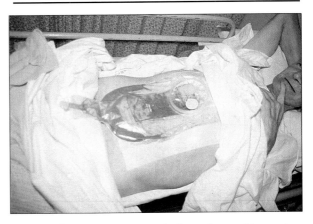

Fig. 406 This patient needed 27 days of intensive care because he developed peritonitis and septicaemia from a small bowel perforation. He subsequently developed a fistula. This needed long-term TPN.

Table 27 Multiple biochemical disturbances

General intensive care Clinical details: Chronic sepsis, TPN	Specimen type: Serum		
Total protein	51	g/l	(60–80)
Albumin	23	g/l	(38–48)
Total calcium	1.79	mmol/l	(2.12–2.55)
Phosphate	1.19	mmol/l	(0.65–1.3)
Bilirubin	40	µmol/l	(<17)
Alkaline phosphatase	289	IU/L	(35–115)
Alanine transaminase	43	IU/L	(0–45)
Sodium	141	mmol/l	(134–147)
Potassium	3.5	mmol/l	(3.4–5.0)
Creatinine	65	µmol/l	(65–110)
Ionised calcium	1.03	mmol/l	(1.19–1.37)
Ionised calcium (corr to pH 7.4)	1.06	mmol/l	(1.19–1.37)
Magnesium	0.69	mmol/l	(0.7–1.0)

This patient's values are abnormal. The patient is on TPN and these deficiencies, notably the plasma calcium, will gradually resolve with changes to the feeding regimen. Magnesium deficiency is rare in isolation; it should always be suspected in patients with hypokalaemia or hypocalcaemia. There is also evidence of obstructive hepatic dysfunction, probably due to cholangitis.

ELECTROPHORESIS

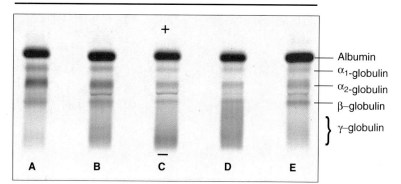

Column A: Acute inflammation; increased α_1 and α_2 bands
Column B: Chronic inflammation; increased α_1, α_2 and
            γ bands
Column C: Polyclonal gammopathy — this pattern is seen in
            chronic inflammation
Column D: Hepatic cirrhosis; β–γ band fusion
Column E: Normal serum

Fig. 407 A semi-quantitative test for serum proteins. There are distinct bands for albumin, α_1- and α_2-globulins, β-globulins and γ-globulins, shown top to bottom.

ELECTROLYTE ABNORMALITIES

Ill patients will often have disturbances of sodium and potassium balance. Less frequently monitored are calcium, magnesium and zinc but these are likely to be disturbed in complex cases as well.

HIGH SODIUM

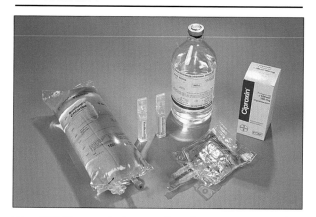

Fig. 408 Many solutions and antibiotics contain a lot of sodium. it is easy to exceed daily requirements of 1–2 mmol/kg per day.

LOW SODIUM

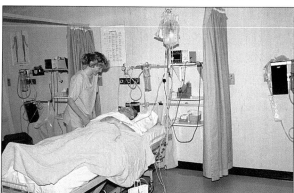

Fig. 409 Dilutional hyponatraemia is often missed and misleading. Another cause illustrated here is irrigation after prostatectomy. This can result in excessive water absorption which in turn may lead to epileptic fits.

Table 28 Common causes of sodium disturbance in the ICU

Normal range: 134–147 mmol/l

High sodium		Low sodium	
Cause	**Example**	**Cause**	**Example**
Excess Na	Intake	Loss Na	Vomiting
	Steroids		Diarrhoea
			Burns
			Diuretics
Water loss	Fever		
	Diuresis	Dilutional	Water overload
	Diarrhoea		Renal failure
			Inappropriate ADH

LOW POTASSIUM

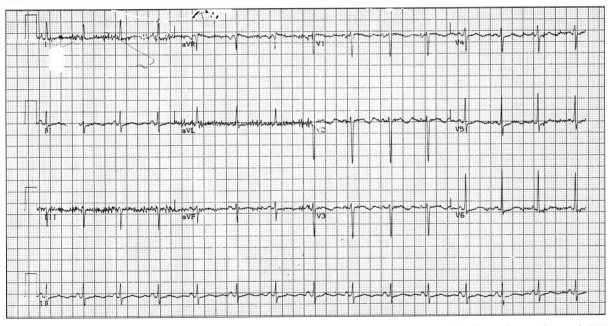

Fig. 410 This ECG shows a small amplitude trace, a decrease in T wave amplitude and a prolonged QT interval. A double hump of the T wave followed by the U wave is characteristic. The serum potassium was 2.2 mmol/l. The clinical features are of weakness and hypotension and cardiac arrest.

HIGH POTASSIUM: PREDIALYSIS

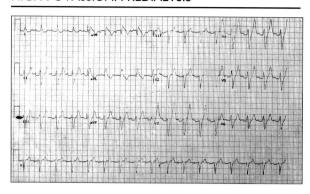

Fig. 411 The characteristic ECG changes of severe hyperkalaemia. There is peaking of the T wave, widening of the QRS complex and disappearance of the P wave as the potassium exceeds 8 mmol/l, as in this case.

POSTDIALYSIS

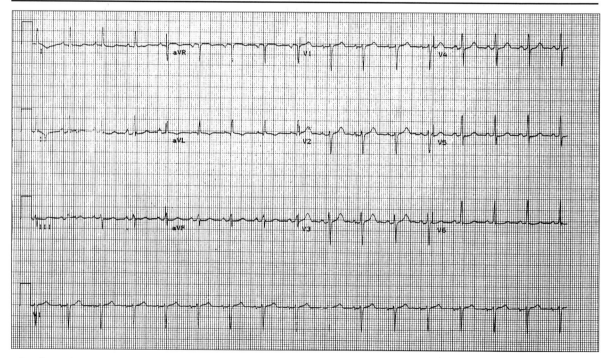

Fig. 412 The patient received 50 ml of 8.47% sodium bicarbonate and 10 ml of 10% calcium gluconate immediately. A glucose and insulin infusion was started. Dialysis was introduced with safe recovery.

Table 29 Common causes of potassium disturbance in the ICU

Reference range: 3.4–5.0 mmol/l

Low potassium		High potassium	
Cause	**Example**	**Cause**	**Example**
Artifact	Sample taken near IV infusion	Artifact	Haemolysis
Low intake	Alcoholic Anorexia	High intake	Sample taken near IV infusion
Excess loss	Gut: Vomiting Diarrhoea Fistula Renal: Diuretic Aldosteronism	Deceased loss	Renal failure Tissue necrosis: Burn Crush injury
Alkalosis		Acidosis	

HYPERCALCAEMIA: THYROID AND PARATHYROID SCAN

Fig. 413 A subtraction image shows persistent residual uptake in the entire left thyroid lobe. An ultrasound was required to establish this in fact was a parathyroid gland that was behind the thyroid gland.

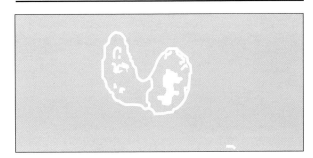

HYPERCALCAEMIA: BIOCHEMISTRY

Table 30 Hypercalcaemia biochemistry

Measurement	Value	Range
Ionised calcium	5.08 mmol/l	1.19–1.37
Parathyroid hormone	1000 pmol/l	29–85

This patient has hyperparathyroidism due to tumour.

Plasma calcium is misleading, as 30–45% is bound to albumin. If the plasma concentration of albumin is low then the total concentration of calcium will also be low. However, the unbound (free or ionised) concentration may be normal, high or low.

A 44-year-old man presented with headaches, dizziness and vomiting for ten days (see **Table 30**). He was unable to drink. He suffered two cardiac arrests caused by VT. To treat his hypercalcaemia he was given a saline infusion, hydrocortisone and calcitonin. His ionised calcium 24 hours later had decreased to 2.63 mmol/l.

HYPOCALCAEMIA

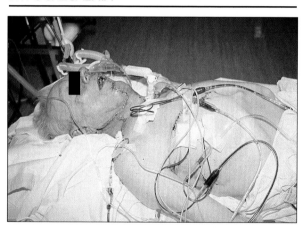

Fig. 414 Radical neck surgery resulting in parathyroid removal, as shown here, and acute renal failure are the two important causes of significant hypocalcaemia in the ICU. Massive blood transfusion can sometimes cause this problem. The anticoagulant (citrate) binds free calcium, inactivating it.

TRACE METAL DEFICIENCIES

Table 31 Trace metal deficiencies

Magnesium	0.58	mmol/l (normal 0.70–1.00)
Copper	9	µmol/l (normal 11–25)
Zinc	5	µmol/l (normal 8–24)

An 80-year-old was admitted in a confused state. She had had diarrhoea for some days with abdominal pain. There were no gross abnormalities on examination. This is probably nutritional.

JAUNDICE

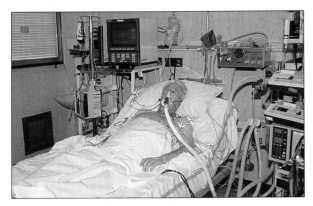

Fig. 415 An obviously jaundiced patient will have a standard series of tests, consisting of plasma bilirubin, albumin, and certain tests of enzyme activity including aspartate or alanine aminotransferase (AST/ALT) and alkaline phosphatase. Increased transaminases are nonspecific indicators of liver damage. Alkaline phosphatase is specific for enzyme induction and grossly increased in cholestasis. Coagulation defects are usual and the prothrombin time is routinely measured as well, as is the blood glucose.

ULTRASOUND OF LIVER

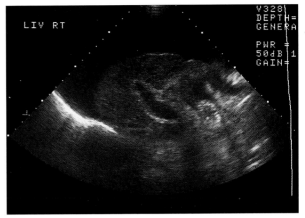

Fig. 416 This ultrasound shows a cirrhotic liver with a large amount of ascites.

LIVER BIOPSY

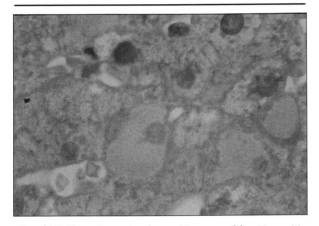

Fig. 417 Chronic active hepatitis caused by Hepatitis B infection. There is cellular infiltration with progressive destruction of the liver parenchyma. 'Ground glass' cells in the centre and right of the biopsy contain an eosinophilic deposit of surface antigen HBsAg.

HEPATITIS MARKERS

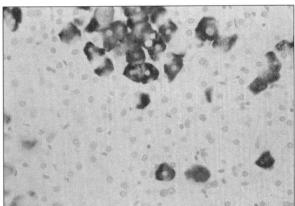

Fig. 418 The cells are hepatitis surface antigen positive. The nucleus appears clear. In core antigen-positive patients the reverse pattern is seen, notably a dark nucleus with a pale surrounding surface. A special stain has been used.

LIVER FUNCTION TESTS 1

Chronic active hepatitis (**Table 32**): markedly increased bilirubin with aminotransferase activity. The pattern of enzyme activity is useful in following the progression of the disease.

Table 32 Liver function tests I: chronic active hepatitis

	64 g/l	37 g/l	2.23 mmol/l	1.04 mmol/l	91 µmol/l	93 IU/l (37°C)	54 IU/l (37°C)
NORMAL ADULT REFERENCE RANGE	TOTAL PROTEIN (60–80)	ALBUMIN (38–48)	CALCIUM (2.12–2.55)	PHOSPHATE (0.65–1.30)	TOTAL BILIRUBIN (<17)	ALK. PHOS (35–115)	AST. (0–45)

LIVER FUNCTION TESTS 2

Cholestatis (**Table 33**): increased bilirubin and raised alkaline phosphatase activity. The clotting screen also shows a prolonged prothrombin time.

Table 33 Liver function tests II: cholestatic activity and clotting screen

General intensive care
Clinical details:
Liver disease

Specimen type: Serum

Cholestatic activity:

Sodium	134	mmol/l	(normal 134–147)
Potassium	3.8	mmol/l	(3.4–5.0)
Total CO$_2$	29	mmol/l	(22–29)
Urea	4.1	mmol/l	(2.5–7.0)
Creatinine	106	µmol/l	(65–110)
Total protein	62	g/l	(60–80)
Albumin	29*	g/l	(38–48)
Bilirubin	274*	µmol/l	(0–17)
Alkaline phosphatase	261*	IU/L	(35–115)
Alanine transaminase	38	IU/L	(0–45)

Clotting screen

Prothrombin time	22	seconds	(13–14)
Kaolin cephalin time	41	seconds	(30–38)
Thrombin time	22	seconds	(15–19)
Plasma fibrinogen	1.6	g/l	(2.0–4.0)
D. Dimer	<0.5	mg/l	(<0.5 mg/l)

CT PANCREAS: OBSTRUCTIVE JAUNDICE

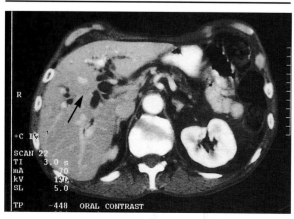

Fig. 419 Carcinoma of the head of pancreas causing obstructive jaundice is shown here by the grossly dilated biliary tree (arrow).

GLUCOSE ABNORMALITIES

Diabetes mellitus is a disorder of glucose metabolism. The classification of the disease may be divided into two main types, an insulin-dependent group (type 1) or non-insulin-dependent group (type 2), which have different causes and treatment regimens. The chronic hyperglycaemia that results produces many systemic changes notably in the eye, the vascular system, the kidney and neurological systems.

BLOOD GLUCOSE

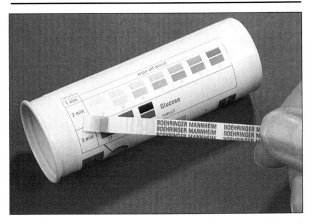

Fig. 420 A simple bedside test can determine blood glucose. The fasting normal is between 3 and 5 mmol/l. All patients in ICU should have their blood glucose estimated regularly since abnormalities are common.

Fig. 422 This patient has a blood glucose of 17 mmol/l. He is not diabetic. In severe injury the catabolic response producing hormones including adrenaline, cortisol and glucagon lead to a 'diabetic-like' state because of insulin resistance. Certain drugs (notably the use of steroids, salbutamol and loop diuretics), TPN, and chronic pancreatitis also produce a secondary diabetes.

HYPOGLYCAEMIA COMA

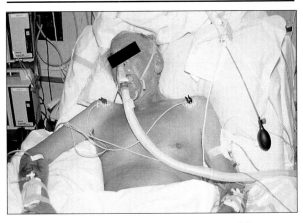

Fig. 421 Blood glucose less than 2 mmol/l. Severe liver disease, malnutrition, pancreatitis and adrenal insufficiency are causes to be remembered in the critically ill.

SECONDARY HYPERGLYCAEMIA

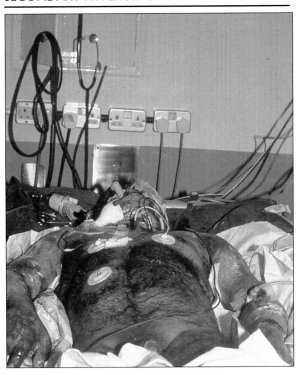

DIABETIC KETOACIDOSIS

A 32-year-old insulin-dependent diabetic developed vomiting and diarrhoea. He was wrongly told not to take insulin.

As shown in **Table 34**, he was severely dehydrated (Haematocrit = 49%) with a life-threatening metabolic acidosis (pH = 6.92 (H^+ = 120 nmol/l), bicarbonate = 2 mmol/l) and compensatory hyperventilation ($PaCO_2$ = 1.6 kPa). He was given saline, insulin and sodium bicarbonate and made a full recovery.

Table 34 Diabetic ketoacidosis

pH (H^+)	6.92 (120 nmol/l)
$PaCO_2$	1.6 kPa
PaO_2	19 kPa
Bicarbonate	2 mmol/l
Base excess	−28 mmol/l
Sodium	127 mmol/l
Potassium	6.4 mmol/l
Urea	8 mmol/l
Blood glucose	31.8 mmol/l
Haemoglobin	16.3 g/dl
White blood cell count	23.7 × 10⁹/l
Haematocrit	49%
Platelets	362 × 10⁹/l

RENAL DISEASE

Renal failure in the critically ill patient is a major cause of concern; even with treatment, there is a mortality of around 50%. Acute renal failure may be potentially reversible with adequate resuscitation. It may complicate pre-existing chronic renal disease or follow obstruction to the urinary tract. The diagnosis should always be considered in every patient entering ICU since it is usually treatable.

Patients commonly present with oliguria (<1 ml/kg/hr). If it is caused by prerenal failure it is usually treatable, usually by a fluid challenge or improving cardiac output. The careful monitoring of potassium (see **Table 29**, p. 125), acidosis and fluid balance is important for safe management. Dopamine in low dosage can improve renal blood flow and should be given (2–5 µg/kg/min).

In established renal failure, renal replacement therapy is indicated (see Chapter 1). The diagnosis is confirmed by finding a urinary sodium >20 mmol/l and a urinary osmolality <350 mmol/kg. A polyuric phase may occur, permitting much easier fluid balance, with a mortality of 35%.

TESTING URINE

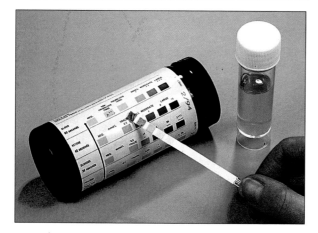

Fig. 423 Ward testing will reveal blood, albumin and glucose.

EXAMINATION OF THE URINE

Table 35 Examination of the urine

Test	Reason
Appearance	Content—see **Table 36**
LABSTIX	
Albumin	Renal disease
Sugar	Diabetes
pH	Acidity
Laboratory	
Osmolality	Concentrating ability
Sodium	Excretory capability
Creatinine clearance	Renal function
Microscopy	
Red blood cells	Glomerulonephritis
	Tumour/infection
White blood cells	Infection
Casts	Renal disease

GREEN URINE DUE TO PROPOFOL

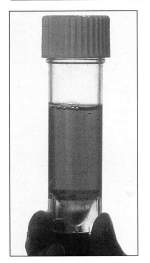

Fig. 424 Coloration caused by propofol.

ORANGE URINE DUE TO RIFAMPICIN

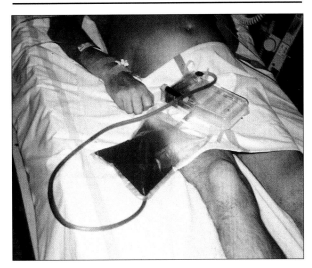

Fig. 425 Coloration caused by rifampicin.

Table 36 Urine colours

Brown	Red	Green	Orange
Blood	Blood	Propofol	Rifampicin
Melanin	Porphyria		Bile

Table 37 Common causes of acute renal failure

Prerenal	Renal	Postrenal
Hypovolaemia	Drugs/nephrotoxins	Obstructive nephropathy
Hypoxia	Haemolysis	
Sepsis	Rhabdomyolysis	
Low cardiac output state	Vascular	
	Glomerulonephritis	
	Chronic pyelonephritis	
	Obstetric	

Routine screening includes measuring plasma concentrations of creatinine and urea. Plasma creatinine remains unchanged throughout adult life and correlates well with glomerular filtration rate. It is a useful screening test to detect early renal impairment. The plasma urea is less precise as a test of renal function because other conditions, such as trauma and haematoma, can increase it.

Fig. 426 A compound fracture of the tibia resulting in hypovolaemic shock. Adequate resuscitation should reverse this situation.

PRERENAL FAILURE

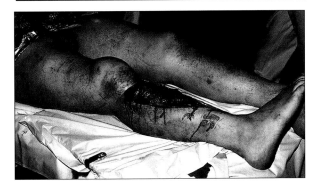

INTRINSIC RENAL DISEASE: GLOMERULONEPHRITIS

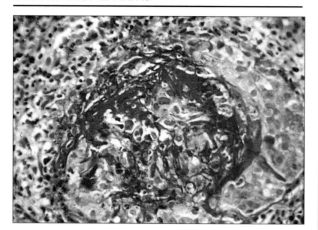

Fig. 427 This renal biopsy shows proliferation of the inflammatory glomeruli epithelial cells to fill the capsular space, which adhere together to produce crescents in 80% or more of the glomeruli.

OBSTRUCTIVE NEPHROPATHY

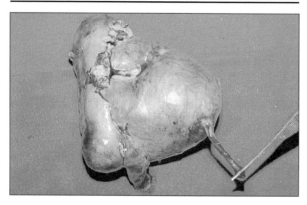

Fig. 429 Pelvo-ureteric obstruction. It is important to exclude these conditions.

RENAL FUNCTION TESTS: MILD IMPAIRMENT

Typical changes after aortic aneurysm surgery are shown in **Table 38**. The high urea reflects some haematoma breakdown as well as renal impairment.

Table 38 Clinical details of mild renal impairment

	Specimen type: Serum		
Sodium	152*	mmol/l	(134–147)
Potassium	3.6	mmol/l	(3.4–5.0)
Urea	17.9*	mmol/l	(2.5–7)
Creatinine	128*	µmol/l	(65–110)

BILATERAL HYDRONEPHROSIS

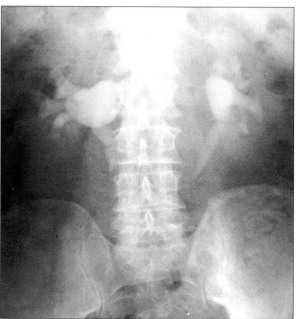

Fig. 428 This intravenous pyelogram shows grossly distended renal pelvices. The cause was an inflammatory aortic aneurysm.

RENAL FUNCTION TESTS: CHRONIC RENAL FAILURE

High creatinine and urea are found despite regular dialysis (**Table 39**). The serum phosphate is characteristically increased, but the plasma calcium can vary from low to high.

Table 39 Clinical details of chronic renal failure

	Specimen type: Serum		
Total protein	63	g/l	(60–80)
Albumin	36	g/l	(38–48)
Total calcium	2.33	mmol/l	(2.12–2.55)
Phosphate	2.18	mmol/l	(0.65–1.30)
Bilirubin	8	µmol/l	(S–17)
Alkaline phospatase	76	IU/l	(35–115)
Alanine transaminase	14	IUl/l	(0–45)
Sodium	139	mmol/l	(134–147)
Potassium	4.4	mmol/l	(3.4–5.0)
Urea	39.0*	mmol/l	(2.5–7.0)
Creatinine	1038*	µmol/l	(65–110)

INFREQUENT ENDOCRINE DISORDERS

ADRENAL HYPOFUNCTION: OMISSION OF STEROID COVER

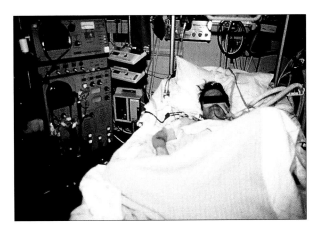

Fig. 430 This man failed to recover consciousness after operation. He was hypotensive and remained so until hydrocortisone was given. Steroids had been tailed off two months before surgery. A short Synacthen test revealed a basal cortisol level of 115 nmol/l (normal range 145–610 nmol/l), increasing to 130 nmol/l at 45 min. A value of >1,000 nmol/l is usually seen in critically ill patients. Infarction or haemorrhage into the adrenal gland in shock or sepsis needs to be considered in hypotensive patients. This condition is probably under-diagnosed.

PRIMARY ADRENAL INSUFFICIENCY: ADDISON'S DISEASE

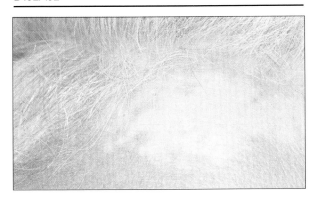

Fig. 431 Vitiligo and hair loss are striking features of Addison's disease where most other skin areas exhibit increased pigmentation. The classic electrolyte changes are a low serum sodium and glucose with a high serum urea and potassium. Muscle cramps, dehydration and hypotension are other features.

MYXOEDEMA

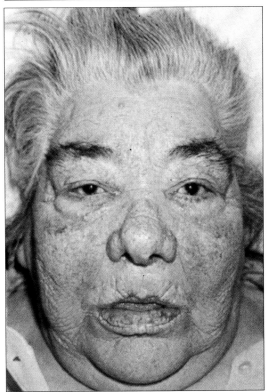

Fig. 432 Non-pitting puffiness of the face, coarsening of the features and uncontrollable hair. Likely to be missed in the ICU but the combination of hypothermia, hypotension, hypoglycaemia and hyponatraemia is so unusual that the clinician should think of this condition.

CENTRAL NERVOUS SYSTEM INFECTIONS

CEREBROSPINAL FLUID (CSF)

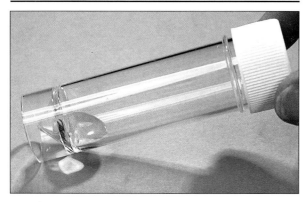

Fig. 433 In the ICU the possibility of infections of the central nervous system must be borne in mind. The normal CSF is colourless and clear. Cloudiness is caused by white cells or organisms. A lumbar puncture should not be attempted in the presence of papilloedema or raised intracranial pressure.

GRAM STAIN: *CRYPTOCOCCUS NEOFORMANS* IN CSF

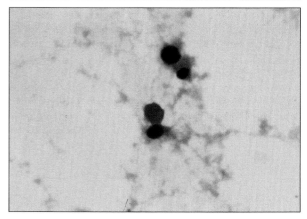

Fig. 434 A most serious and lethal complication of *Cryptococcus pneumonia* is meningoencephalitis, and is a frequent infection in AIDS. This fungal infection is worldwide and thought to be spread by bird droppings. Many other commoner organisms can cause life-threatening meningitis such as *Meningococcal meningitis.*

TUBERCULOUS MENINGITIS

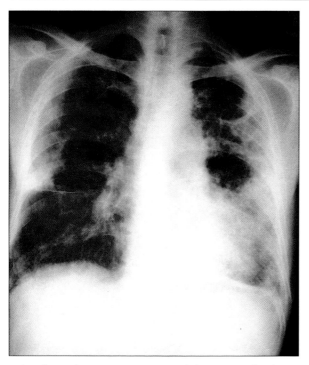

Fig. 435 This cavitating apical lesion in the lung raised the possibility of tuberculosis in a 43-year-old patient with chronic renal failure.

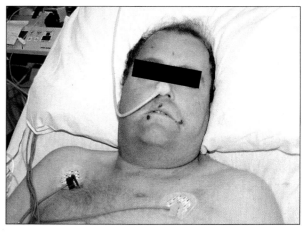

Fig. 436 This patient developed a progressive loss of consciousness. A lumbar puncture revealed a slightly turbid fluid under pressure. Subsequent culture supported the diagnosis of tuberculosis. He has herpes simplex around the mouth as well.

CONTENT OF NORMAL CSF

Table 40

	Appearance	Pressure	Glucose	Protein	Cells
Normal	Crystal clear	80-200 mm Hg	3.5 mmol/l	15-45 mg/l	0.5 lymphocytes
Traumatic tap	Bloodstained	Normal	Increased	Red cells	
Subarachnoid haemorrhage	Bloody	Increased	Normal	Increased	Red cells
Bacterial meningitis	Turbid	Increased	Low	Increased	Neutrophils++
Viral meningitis	Clear	Increased	Normal	Normal	Lymphocytes++
TB meningitis	Opalescent	Increased	Low	Increased	Lymphocytes++

HAEMATOLOGY

The investigation of clotting abnormalities is a major part of the work in the ICU. Drug-induced effects and nutritional deficiency are also seen.

THROMBOELASTOGRAPH

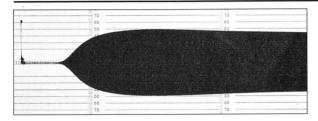

Fig. 437 A normal example from a liver transplant operation. Understanding the complex process of clotting can be aided by the thromboelastograph.

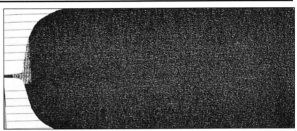

Fig. 438 Hypercoagulable states produce a short line with a very wide body.

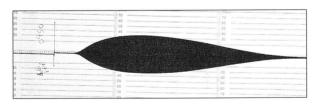

Fig. 439 Fibrinolysis leads to a 'fish' with a long hook and narrow body.

DISSEMINATED COAGULATION SYNDROME

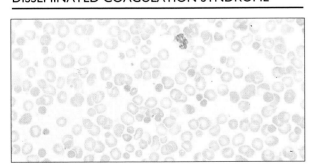

Fig. 440 Blood picture shows few platelets and microspheres typical of DIC. From a patient with 80% burns.

BLOOD TRANSFUSION REACTION

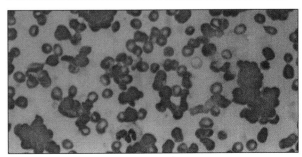

Fig. 441 Cold agglutinins after major blood mismatch reaction. Hypotension and renal failure followed.

FOLATE DEFICIENCY

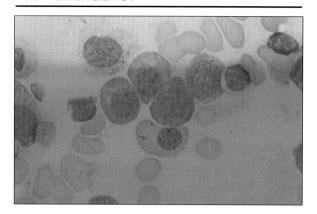

Fig. 442 Megaloblastic bone marrow due to folate deficiency. Precipitous decreases in folate are seen in ICU patients and are likely to be forgotten about. Replacement should be given to all patients seriously ill for more than two or three days. It should also be given after anaesthesia lasting more than two hours when nitrous oxide has been given.

SICKLE CELL CRISIS: SICKLE CELL PREPARATION

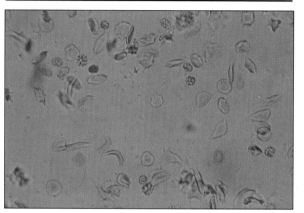

Fig. 443 Patients with haemoglobin SS, which occurs in 1:1000 of blacks, can develop a painful and life-threatening crisis precipitated by dehydration, hypoxia or acidosis.

APLASTIC BONE MARROW

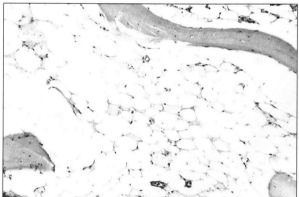

Fig. 444 The architecture remains but fat replaces the normal haemopoetic cells. Drugs are usually the cause; these include: antibiotics, tranquillisers, anti-thyroid and anti-diabetic drugs, anti-rheumatics, anticonvulsants and antimitotic agents.

MICROBIOLOGY

ICU units around the world now have encountered the problems of emergence strains of organisms. Proper laboratory expertise and microbiological advice on prescribing, surveillance of the ICU infection rate and an overall epidermiological supervision of the hospital is a requirement for safe practice.

SETTLE PLATES

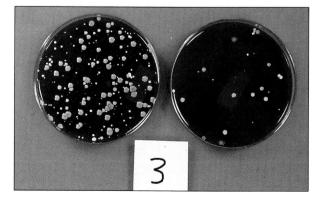

Fig. 445 The bacterial count in the ICU on agar plates showing before (right) and after (left) the ward round.

METHICILLIN-RESISTANT *STAPHYLOCOCCUS AUREUS:* (MRSA)

Fig. 446 Patients being transferred between hospitals may result in a hospital epidemic of MRSA and all such cases should be isolated in a side ward until micro-biological clear-ance.

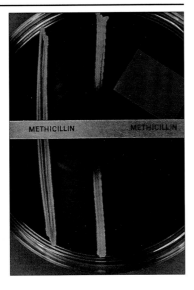

MULTIPLE-RESISTANT *KLEBSIELLA* PNEUMONIA

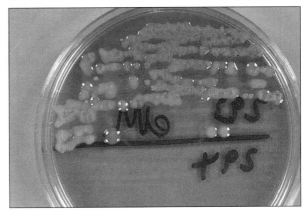

Fig. 447 Repatriated patients may also transfer resistant organisms and need screening.

PSEUDOMONAS AERUGINOSA OUTBREAK

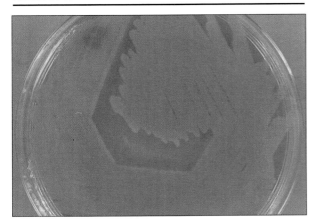

Fig. 448 The single most important factor in ICU and ward cross-infection is the failure of the staff, especially medical personnel, to wash their hands after dealing with an individual patient.

ANTIBIOTIC SELECTION

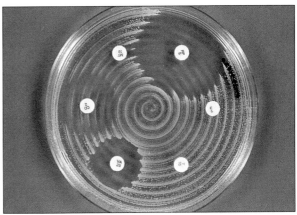

Fig. 449 The use of antibiotic discs to determine the antibiotic susceptibility of any given organism cultured.

Fig. 450 Risus sardonicus facies due to *Clostridia tetani* infection. The spore-bearing organism is found in the soil, and infection can occur due to soil contamination of a wound. Farmers, athletes and road traffic accident victims are likely to be infected in this way. The development of muscle spasms presents as jaw stiffness, and spasms of the facial muscles give rise to this characteristic grin. The spasms become generalised and often triggered by noise and autonomic lability develops. Severe cases will require debridement of wounds, human tetanus immunoglobulin, penicillin, diazepam and ven-tilation in the ICU. Recovery is inversely proportional to incubation time.

TETANUS

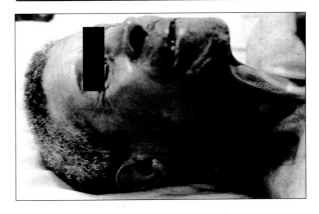

LIST OF ABBREVIATIONS

AIDS	Acquired immune deficiency syndrome
ARDS	Adult (acute) respiratory distress syndrome
ATLS	Advanced trauma life support course
$A\bar{v}DO_2$	Arterio-mixed venous oxygen difference
AVG	Average
BSA	Body surface area
CaO_2	Content of oxygen in arterial blood
CMV	Continuous mandatory ventilation
CO	Cardiac output
CO Hb	Carboxyhaemoglobin
COPD	Chronic obstructive airways disease
CPAP	Continuous positive airway pressure
CPR	Cardiopulmonary resuscitation
CSF	Cerebrospinal fluid
CT	Computerised tomography
$C\bar{v}O_2$	Content of oxygen in mixed venous blood
CVP	Central venous pressure
DIC	Disseminated intravascular coagulation
DO_2I	Delivery of oxygen
ECMO	Extracorporeal membrane oxygenation
FEV_1	Forced expiratory volume in 1 second
F_IO_2	Inspired oxygen concentration
FRC	Functional residual capacity
FVC	Forced vital capacity
Hb	Haemoglobin
HGB	Haemoglobin
ICP	Intracranial pressure
ICU	Intensive care unit
IPPV	Intermittent positive pressure ventilation
MAP	Mean arterial pressure
MI	Myocardial infarction
MPA	Mean pulmonary arterial pressure
MPAP	Mean pulmonary artery pressure
O_2	Oxygen
PAC	Pulmonary artery catheter
$PaCO_2$	Carbon dioxide pressure
PaO_2	Arterial oxygen pressure
PCA	Patient controlled analgesia
PCWP	Pulmonary artery 'wedge' pressure
PEEP	Positive end expiratory pressure
PVR	Pulmonary vascular resistance
RR	Respiratory rate
SaO_2	Arterial oxygen saturation
SBE	Subacute bacterial endocarditis
$SvCO_2$	Venous (mixed) oxygen saturation
$S\bar{v}O_2$	Mixed venous oxygen saturation
SVR	Systemic vascular resistance
SVRI	Systemic vascular resistance
TPN	Total perenteral nutrition
Tv	Tidal volume
Vc	Vital capacity
VO_2I	Oxygen consumption indexed to body surface area

INDEX